D1648129

# NATURAL THERAPIES FOR PARKINSON'S DISEASE

# NATURAL THERAPIES FOR PARKINSON'S DISEASE

### Dr. Laurie K. Mischley

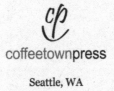

coffeetownpress

Seattle, WA

Published by Coffeetown Press
PO Box 95462
Seattle, WA 98145

Cover design by Sabrina Sun

Contact: info@Coffeetownpress.com

ISBN: 978-60381-043-2 (Paper)
ISBN: 978-1-60381-015-9 (Case)

There are three truths in science.
First, they say it isn't true.
Then, they say it's true, but not important.
Finally, they say it is true and important, but not new.

—Anonymous


The person who says it cannot be done should not interrupt the person doing it.

—Chinese Proverb

# Contents

# Introduction

This book is intended to be the first of several editions. It can be used as a resource by patients, physicians, caregivers, and relatives of those with Parkinsonism. It is not a thorough or comprehensive overview of Parkinsonism but a glimpse of how one might look at the disease from alternative perspectives.

There are over 1.5 million people in the US with Parkinson's disease, and many of them are currently using some form of alternative medicine. Neurologists are largely uneducated about complementary therapies, and patients, who are typically elderly and reliant on Medicare, lack the resources to consult with a qualified practitioner.

I do not propose to have the solution for Parkinson's disease (PD). I do believe that the information on the following pages is valuable to those looking to discourage the disease.
This book is unique in that it is just as valuable to individuals with PD as it is to their children, a high-risk and often neglected group.

I do not believe the solution is to purchase or enact all of the items on the pages that follow. Each individual's process is different; and different bodies have different needs.

This is book is intended to be *integrative* you don't need to choose between conventional and alternative medicine. The concurrent use of pharmaceutical therapies for relief of symptoms is highly recommended.

That said, these pages are filled with recommendations that have not been completely investigated for efficacy. Recommendations included were chosen because I understand them to have therapeutic potential. They are relatively easy to implement, and I believe that for some, the benefits clearly outweigh the risks. My primary intention is to increase the reader's awareness of non-conventional therapeutic options and catalyze interdisciplinary communication and collaboration.

Be well,


Laurie K Mischley, ND

# I. How to Use This Book

This book is designed as an easily accessed reference manual. Turn to a particular chapter if you have a question, or read it cover-to-cover.

## *Whose questions are in italics?*

The questions in italics are reflective of those I've been asked by hundreds of patients with Parkinsonism over the years. The format was chosen to serve those with the disease who do not have access to a physician specializing in complementary and alternative medicine in Parkinson's disease.

## *How do I know which therapies to use?*

All individuals with Parkinsonism are different and thus require different therapies to manage their disease. Resources, symptoms, and community support further dictate which therapies should be considered.

Highlight or dog-ear pages you're interested in pursuing and bring them up with your doctor.

➔ Recommendation for Action.

The arrow denotes the author's recommendation for intervention. It is set apart from the rest of the text for two reasons:

1.  Ease of use. If you don't really care about why the recommendations are being made, you can easily flip through the pages and simply see what is being recommended.

2.  The recommendations denoted with the arrow are considered "premature" according to those basing their decisions on controlled clinical trials.

---

## DOC BOX

Text in a **DOC BOX** is intended for those curious about pathophysiology or mechanism of action. It's information to take to your doctor.

---

# Why recommend therapies without the support of controlled clinical trials?

Ideally, one wouldn't. But we don't live in an ideal world. Research is expensive and takes many, many years to complete. One must balance scientific scrutiny with common sense.

For instance, consumption of coffee and tea has been shown to protect against PD. Say you are a 40 year old man, you have always had a problem with constipation, and you have a father with PD. You can wait a couple decades for a double-blind placebo-controlled trial costing millions of dollars to ask the question, "Will tea or coffee consumption throughout life decrease PD in those with a family history of the disease?" Or, you can evaluate the information we do have today and decide for yourself whether the potential benefits outweigh the potential risks. Alternatively, you can just:

→ Drink tea or coffee regularly.

# II. WHAT CAUSES PARKINSONISM?

## What is Parkinsonism?

Parkinsonism is a disorder of movement. It is defined by the following symptoms:
- Slowness
- Rigidity
- Resting tremor
- Unstable posture

One does not need to have all of the symptoms to qualify for a diagnosis or to have a disease process underway.

## What causes Parkinsonism?

Most likely, it is caused by a combination of genetic and environmental factors.

Predisposing genes and various environmental factors differ among individuals, making it difficult to find one culprit.

## What can we do about it?

If you want to change the equation, you have to change the variables.

**PD = Genes + Environment**

The solution:

1. Identify those with the predisposition
2. Encourage a protective environment

# TERMINOLOGY

## *What's the difference between Parkinson's disease and Parkinsonism?*

Conventionally, Parkinsonism is a general term, while PD denotes a specific disease. For the purposes of this book, the terms are used interchangeably. Both terms will be used to describe the occurrence of the following symptoms: slowness, rigidity, tremor, and postural instability.

Below is the currently accepted differential diagnosis of parkinsonian symptoms.[1] Perhaps most unfortunate is that a 2009 review of PD in the elite journal *Neurology* references this 1992 algorithm, suggesting there has been no shift in how we view Parkinsonism in 17 years![2]

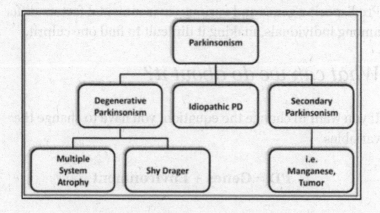

## What is Idiopathic Parkinson's disease?

The term *idiopathic* designates a disease having no known cause. The name concedes our ignorance about how these symptoms came to be.

One can develop a tremor and slowness in several ways, including manganese exposure, MPTP, and trauma to a specific part of the brain. Idiopathic PD is a term reserved for individuals with the cardinal symptoms of PD but with no obvious cause of the symptoms.

Idiopathic Parkinson's disease is an unfortunate name for a disease so desperately yearning for a cure. The term *idiopathic* forces affected individuals and their doctors to identify with a disease that, by definition, is not understood.

## Why are so many people's symptoms dismissed as "idiopathic?"

Some conditions lend themselves well to study. Those involving the brain do not.

Brain biopsies are, for the time being, impractical. Furthermore, dopamine is but one of a dozen brain chemicals affected in Parkinsonism. These chemicals not only affect the brain, but also the endocrine, gastro-intestinal, skeletal-muscular, and emotional systems as well.

## Once the diagnosis becomes clear, why don't doctors go looking for the cause?

In short, because there is no proof (double-blind placebo-controlled studies) that changing things now will impact the course of your disease.

Unless the line of inquiry will result in useful information and improvement in a disease, most doctors shy away from these questions.

It's not that the studies are negative. The studies have not been done! No study has ever asked this fundamental question:

# What causes Parkinsonism?

Assuming the goal is a cure, the task at hand is identifying the cause. The closer we get to answering this question, the closer we get to closing this chapter of history.

# PATHOPHYSIOLOGY

Pathophysiology is the study of the mechanics of dysfunction. It is what we see in those with disease, as compared to those without disease. Studying pathophysiology often provides insight into disease processes and opens the doors to new therapeutics.

## LEWY BODIES

Lewy bodies are found in the cytoplasm of neurons in patients with PD. They are the hallmark of the disease.

## What are they? Where are they found?

If we look at the brain of an individual with Parkinson's disease, we will see Lewy bodies. They are found floating in the cytoplasm of neurons.

## What is a Lewy body?

Lewy bodies are composed of α-synuclein and ubiquitin, two proteins associated with disease progression in PD.

## Are Lewy bodies bad?

Not necessarily. In fact, they may actually be reflective of a protective response in the brain. They may be one of the mechanisms by which our brain clears harmful proteins, such as α-synuclein.

## Are Lewy bodies seen in other diseases?

Yes. In addition to PD, they are seen in dementia (with and without Parkinsonian symptoms), Down syndrome, infantile neuroaxonal dystrophy, and several others.

Approximately 30% of elderly individuals without neurological symptoms have Lewy bodies. Their presence doesn't necessarily equate disease.[3]

## What is the role of Lewy bodies?

They are probably an aggresome intended to facilitate the clearance of misfolded, accumulated proteins, such as α-synuclein.[4]

## ALPHA-SYNUCLEIN (α-synuclein)

α-Synuclein is a protein that accumulates in diseased neurons in PD.

## *Can α-synuclein predict PD?*

Probably not. Measuring α-synuclein isn't easy—brain biopsies are difficult, and imaging techniques are not readily available.

Additionally, α-synuclein accumulates in the substantia nigra relatively late in the course of PD.[5]

## *Is there a way to reduce the accumulation of α-synuclein within neurons?*

The ability to degrade accumulated proteins within diseased neurons would revolutionize PD therapeutics. Finding an agent capable of 'unfolding' and dissolving these tangled proteins would offer the first real hope of reversing the disease. Many individuals and companies are aggressively seeking a medicine with this capability.

## *Do any therapies look promising?*

Thus far, only *in vitro* studies have been done. These are studies not done in a living organism, but in a Petri dish or test tube.

Curcumin, a molecule in the common spice turmeric, and beta-carotene, a molecule giving carrots their orange color, are effective *in vitro*.[6,7]

These results are preliminary and it's too soon to tell whether increasing these foods in the diet will improve the course of PD. In the meantime, why *not* drink a bit more carrot juice and cook with a bit more turmeric?

## GENETICS

### *Is there a Parkinson gene?*

More than 10 genes have been identified that are associated with PD. There are several genes that increase an individual's risk of developing PD, some rare and some rather common. Having a PD-related gene doesn't mean you'll get the disease, and you may have a PD gene even if you don't have a family history of PD.

### *Are genetic tests available?*

www.23andme.com is a resource for mapping your genetic code. It is a unique study of PD genetics, where you can have your genes mapped for only $25. It is an excellent resource for individuals with PD and will likely contribute to our understanding about genetics in PD.

## Will my genetic profile shape the way I treat PD?

At this time, treatment of PD is not shaped by your genetic profile.

# III. Reconsidering the Disease Process

## Limitations in Assessment

Some conditions lend themselves well to study. Those involving the brain do not.

Brain biopsies are, for the time being, impractical. Furthermore, dopamine is but one of a dozen brain chemicals affected in Parkinsonism. These chemicals not only affect the brain but also the endocrine, gastro-intestinal, skeletal-muscular, and emotional systems as well.

## *What Causes Parkinsonism?*

Assuming the goal is a cure, the task at hand is identifying the cause. The closer we get to answering, "What causes Parkinsonism?" the closer we get to closing this chapter of history.

So what's the most direct course to understanding how to prevent PD?

Studies suggest that more than 50% of the mass of the substantia nigra has been lost by the time the first symptoms of Parkinsonism appear. Loss of smell and constipation may be early symptoms.

The later in the course of the disease that the symptoms are identified, the more difficult it is to bring the patient change that really matters.

# Why don't we study prevention?

The late onset of Parkinson's symptoms makes it very difficult to study. Researchers estimate the disease process has probably already been underway for a decade by the time the first symptoms appear.

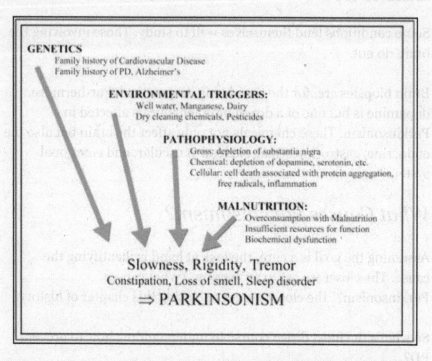

**GENETICS**
Family history of Cardiovascular Disease
Family history of PD, Alzheimer's

**ENVIRONMENTAL TRIGGERS:**
Well water, Manganese, Dairy
Dry cleaning chemicals, Pesticides

**PATHOPHYSIOLOGY:**
Gross: depletion of substantia nigra
Chemical: depletion of dopamine, serotonin, etc.
Cellular: cell death associated with protein aggregation,
free radicals, inflammation

**MALNUTRITION:**
Overconsumption with Malnutrition
Insufficient resources for function
Biochemical dysfunction

Slowness, Rigidity, Tremor
Constipation, Loss of smell, Sleep disorder
⇒ PARKINSONISM

And even if we could predict who will develop PD in 10 years, there is no conventional remedy to offer them. Given the side effects and limitations of dopamine repletion therapy, the available PD medications are useless for any significant amount of prevention.

Parkinsonism is quite a variable disease. I have heard all of the following from my Parkinson's patients over the years:

> "I don't tremor on the outside, but have disruptive tremor in my chest."

"This all started when I slipped and fell."

"This started with an infection in my leg."

"I lost the ability to smell one weekend 20 years ago. I developed restless legs and a sleep disorder, now I have PD."

"I have a family history of "benign tremor'."

"My only symptom is that my chest is being pulled to the ground."

While each one of these patients ended up with a diagnosis of Parkinson's Disease, different factors are probably in play for each of these different people. For the sake of study, convenience, and lack of better diagnostic tools, they are all treated the same. Until we develop an algorithm and a method of differentiation, it will be expensive and time consuming to study prevention.

Let's take one specific example, **manganism**. Manganese toxicity is clinical indistinguishable from PD. Do you know your manganese level? When was the last time it was tested? Only a small percentage of individuals with Parkinsonism have manganese toxicity. For the individual with manganism, this is essential information. But from a public health perspective, it would add significant cost to the health care system to test each person with slowness, rigidity, or tremor for manganese, and thus is not recommended.

## Should everyone with Parkinsonism have a comprehensive evaluation?

However, since we have tools for early detection and physicians

17

with an understanding of environmental and nutritional medicine, it is possible to impart real and positive change. A comprehensive history can guide the evaluation, limiting unnecessary testing: for example, an individual who has never had a gastro-intestinal complaint does not need to be tested for H. pylori.

## *What about the cost of the evaluation?*

**An ounce of prevention is worth a pound of cure.**

—Ben Franklin

The healthcare system in 2010 is deeply broken. We spend the majority of our health care dollars on symptom management, chronic preventable diseases, and end of life care. We therefore have no choice but to shift our focus towards prevention, reducing all of these costs over time.

Pharmaceutical drugs do not offer solutions to the diseases caused by the Western lifestyle. I am not anti-pharmaceutical companies or industry! Pharmaceutical drugs just happen to excel at symptom management, not disease prevention. To truly impart change, resources need to go to the study of epidemiology, environmental medicine, patient education, disease prevention and health promotion.

Only testing that will result in action should be conducted. Don't go on a fishing expedition. Don't be a conspiracy theorist about why you have the symptoms you do. The goal is to understand what is going wrong in a diseased body and take measures to correct it.

# Animal Models

Many animals have unwillingly given their life to the study of Parkinsonism, and for that I am grateful.

Studies of drug addicts, pesticides, and mice have pointed us toward dopamine and the substantia nigra. We now understand a little bit more about protein aggregation, mitochondrial insufficiency, reactive oxygen species (ROS, free radicals), and tissue destruction. Animal models have been invaluable in our understanding of pathophysiology.

But transferring research from bench to bedside is an art. For every study done on animals, we have to translate its applicability to humans, and of course, to our actual patient.

We can give a mouse a chemical that can make it move slowly and have a tremor. We will have no idea what the mouse may be feeling, perceiving, or thinking. It is unlikely that this mouse and the person with Parkinsonism have the same thing going on. We know how to cure this mouse—we prevent it from being exposed to the chemical. But my patient is not a mouse that has been genetically bred and exposed to this chemical.

It's important, therefore, to keep perspective on what can and cannot, be gleaned from animal research.

**Treat the Patient, Not the Disease.**

## What is biochemical individuality?

While PD symptoms are similar from one patient to the next, the factors that contributed to the development of the disease are likely quite different from person to person. For some, genetics plays a strong role. Others may have grown up on farms sprayed heavily with pesticides or been exposed to dry cleaning chemicals. Some individuals are diagnosed in their thirties, others in their 60's. Some may have manganese toxicity that has been misdiagnosed as

Parkinson's disease. Just as each person has a different set of circumstances, the best treatment will vary from person to person.

## How do I go about finding out what is causing my symptoms?

A careful history, screening for known associations with Parkinsonism, is the first place to start. Your provider needs to be familiar with the epidemiology of Parkinson's disease, and keep record of notable associations. Did you work in the dry cleaning operation, or as a farmer spraying pesticides? Did you grow up drinking well water, or living next door to an aluminum factory? Do you have a history of gastric ulcers?

It is your physician's job to understand the mechanism by which each of the above associations is relevant to your Parkinsonism.

## What about using laboratory tests in Parkinsonism?

A comprehensive history can guide the evaluation, limiting unnecessary testing. For example, an individual who has never had gastro-intestinal symptoms does not need to be tested for H. pylori.

Submitting blood, hair, stool, and urine samples is all part of a comprehensive workup. If you have a disease that is negatively impacting your life, for which there is no cure, why leave any stone unturned?

## What about a trial-and-error approach?

Some individuals prefer to play it safe and not experiment with unconventional therapies. Others are reckless and jump on any fad diet or treatment they hear about.

There is no right way to approach Parkinson's disease, no guaranteed formula for success. Know yourself, keep an open mind, and stay informed. Realize that your situation, preferences, and responses are unique to you. With each new treatment you come across, whether alternative or conventional, ask yourself: "What do I have to gain?" "What do I have to lose?"

# IV. Schools of Thought

## a. NATUROPATHIC MEDICINE

### *What is naturopathic medicine?*

Naturopathic medicine was founded on the following philosophic beliefs:
- The Healing Power of Nature
- Identify and Treat the Causes
- First, Do No Harm
- Doctor as Teacher
- Treat the Whole Person
- Prevention
- Wellness

### *What sort of training to naturopathic physicians receive?*

Naturopathic doctors are trained in the art and science of natural healthcare at accredited medical colleges. Naturopathic medical school is a 4-year post-baccalaureate degree, as is conventional medical school.

The curriculum is described as 'eclectic'— NDs study nutritional medicine, herbal medicine, pharmaceutical therapies, Traditional Chinese Medicine, physical medicine, and mind-body medicine, among many other strategies for health. The goal is to know what is available, and help the patient improve their health.

# How is naturopathic medicine different from allopathic medicine?

Allopathic medicine (MD) tends to study disease, and the strength of allopathic medicine is in the management of symptoms.

**MDs play better defense.**

Naturopathic medicine (ND) tends to study health, and the strength of naturopathic medicine is in the prevention and improvement of function.

**NDs play better offense.**

As any sports team requires both a strong offence and defense to be successful. An individual with PD needs both symptom management and optimization of function. Neither is superior to the other, and both perspectives are absolutely necessary to a patient's care.

That these lines are blurring is a great advance in medicine. NDs and MDs are forming partnerships with increasing frequency, and the 'team' approach is thriving in various settings, with providers learning from one another, and patients benefitting!

# Do NDs prescribe pharmaceutical drugs?

Naturopathic physicians are trained to prescribe pharmaceutical drugs. If a pharmaceutical drug is in line with the naturopathic philosophy, yes— pharmaceuticals are prescribed.

# Do all states license naturopathic doctors?

Unfortunately, no. Naturopathic physicians are licensed primary care providers in the following US locations:

- Alaska
- California
- District of Columbia
- Idaho
- Maine
- Montana
- Oregon
- Vermont
- Puerto Rico
- Arizona
- Connecticut
- Hawaii
- Kansas
- Minnesota
- New Hampshire
- Utah
- Washington
- Virgin Islands

NDs are recognized in the Canadian territories:

- British Columbia
- Manitoba
- Ontario
- Saskatchewan

State laws vary regarding insurance reimbursement and scope of practice.

# b. NUTRITIONAL MEDICINE

Nutritional medicine is a method of influencing health, and the course of disease, through the use of diet and nutrients. It is a science practiced by naturopathic doctors (NDs), allopathic doctors (MDs), chiropractors (DCs), nutritionists, and other health care practitioners.

Nutritional medicine dates back to about 400BC, when Hippocrates, the Father of Medicine, said "Let your food be your medicine and your medicine be your food." Hippocrates is credited with being the first physician to challenge the belief that disease was a punishment inflicted by the gods. He rejected the role of divine forces and superstitions in illness and taught instead that disease was the product of diet, environment, and living habits.

Advances in our understanding of anatomy, physiology, and biochemistry have advanced the study of nutritional medicine substantially.

## What is Nutrition?

Contrary to popular belief, nutrition is not the food that we eat. While some foods certainly provide nutrients, nutrition also comes from sunlight, fresh air, water, and even the organisms living within us. Let's start with some definitions.

**Diet**—n. The kinds of foods that a person habitually eats.

**Nutrients**—n. Chemicals needed to live and grow, or a substance used in metabolism which must be taken from the environment. Examples are vitamins, minerals, and accessory nutrients.

**Nutrition**—n. The branch of science that deals with nutrients, the substances that provide nourishment essential for growth and maintenance of life.

Nutrition is about optimizing function. Nutritionists study physiology—how the body functions—and then ask the question, "What can be done to optimize function and keep the system working properly?" While the field of nutrition is often placed in the category of "alternative medicine," it is simply the application of a basic understanding of biochemistry and physiology.

## But I thought that nutrition came from food!?

Food has the potential to be an excellent source of nutrition—kale, nuts, and eggs are great examples. Unfortunately, there are plenty of foods with minimal nutritional value, i.e. corn dogs and ice cream. Interestingly, nutrition comes from several sources besides diet. For instance, vitamin D is derived from sunlight, and vitamin K often comes from the bacteria living in your gut.

## How does nutrition work with conventional medicine?

Nutrition is the study and practice of optimizing function, so in a sense it works with every other discipline. There are no contraindications (negative side effects) for optimizing function. The worst-case scenario is that your system (brain, body, connections between the two) starts working a bit better and your medication dosages need to be adjusted. There should be no

contraindications between any of the recommendations in this book
and those made by your other practitioners.

## Why is nutrition relevant in PD?

The concepts of nutrition are especially pertinent to those living
with PD for several reasons.

- Some foods have been shown to increase or decrease an
  individual's risk of developing PD.

- There is ongoing research on how some nutritional factors
  may slow the progress of the disease and reduce PD
  symptoms.

- The motor complications associated with PD have the
  potential to interfere with feeding, creating difficulties
  unique to this population.

- Individuals with PD seem to have different caloric
  requirements, even before the disease symptoms, than those
  without PD.

- Some of the most commonly used PD medications interfere
  with nutrients.

## Is it possible to change the disease course with nutrition?

We don't know because the research has not been done. Studies
looking at previous intake of foods and nutrients have many
limitations. No researchers have taken two groups of patients with

PD, fed them two different diets, and watched to see if their diseases progressed differently.

## Nutritional issues specific to the elderly

- Vitamin B12 deficiency

  Vitamin B12 deficiency is the most common nutritional
  deficiency of the elderly. A recent study of 800+ patients in
  the neurology department of a hospital revealed that about
  20% of patients were deficient in vitamin B12. Symptoms of
  deficiency included unsteady walking in the darkness and a
  decreased ability to perceive vibration. Deficiency was
  associated with chronic diseases such as high blood
  pressure, coronary heart disease, diabetes, and
  Parkinsonism.[8]

- Decreased intake

  The elderly tend to be less active—which requires fewer
  calories than activity does. Metabolism slows, and people
  literally break down more than they build up.

- Loss of digestive enzymes

  With age, the production of stomach acid, hydrochloric acid
  (HCl) declines. Acidity of gastric contents is a requirement
  for digestion. Loss of this enzyme leads to nutritional
  malabsorption, abnormal growth of gut flora (bugs), and
  reduced motility.

- More time spent indoors

  Being less active overall, the elderly venture out less. When
  they do go out, they tend to avoid becoming "weathered."

29

They tend to stay indoors, reducing their exposure to vitamin D, sourced from sunshine.

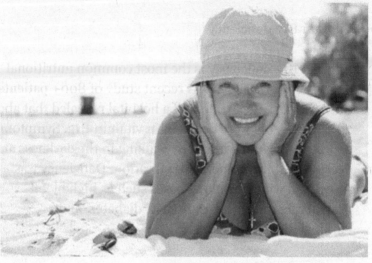

→ Get outdoors more! Expose your skin to the sun—try gardening, or walking outdoors in short shorts and a tank top!

→ Diversify your diet!

Most Americans eat the same 10-20 meals over and over. For all the foods we have access to, the standard American diet is embarrassingly non-varied. When was the last time you had a pomegranate, fava beans, or a good dose of turmeric? (All are recommended for patients with Parkinsonism.)

→ Commit to trying new foods and different presentations of foods you have already tried. Use recipes from the Middle East and Mediterranean, where beans, herbs, and spices are frequently used.

## Nutritional issues specific to Parkinsonism

- Constipation

  Constipation is a well-known complication in Parkinsonism.
  The ability to move food through the digestive tract slows.
  When food starts to 'back up', individuals tend to lose their
  appetite. (See Section entitled: Constipation)

- Movement is difficult

  Non-affected individuals tend to take for granted the ease
  with which they are able to get up, make themselves a quick
  meal, and be on their way. Cooking food from scratch is
  time- and motion-intensive, and thus people with
  Parkinsonism tend to eat more prepared foods, or rely on
  caregivers.

- Vitamin D deficiency

  Vitamin D deficiency is increasingly becoming recognized as
  an epidemic in areas far from the equator and in cultures
  where most time is spent indoors. Individuals with
  Parkinson's disease are at increased risk of vitamin D
  deficiency. (See Section entitled: Vitamin D)

  → Levodopa interferes with absorption and utilization of
    nutrients

  High protein meals can interfere with the absorption of
  levodopa (C/L, Sinemet), causing people to eat more
  carbohydrates and avoid protein. C/L depletes the body of

folic acid and increases the requirement of vitamin B6. (See Section entitled: Drug-Nutrient Interactions)

➔ Medication-related side effects

Dry mouth, nausea, vomiting, loss of appetite, insomnia, fatigue, and anxiety all have the ability to alter nutritional intake.

## Diet and Parkinsonism

# Are there any foods associated with the development of Parkinson's disease?

Dairy has been identified by three large prospective studies that have asked the question, "Is there anything people eat that is associated with an increased development of Parkinson's disease?" (See Section entitled: Dairy)

➔ Avoid all forms of dairy: milk, cream, cheese, yogurt, and ice cream.

➔ Children of individuals with Parkinsonism should avoid these foods whenever possible.

# Are there foods that have been shown to be protective against the development of Parkinson's disease?

A large, prospective study suggested that diets with a high intake of fruit, vegetables, legumes, whole grains, nuts, fish, and poultry were protective against Parkinson's disease. Protection was also associated with low intake of saturated fat and moderate intake of alcohol.[9]

---

**Dietary Guidelines for PD**

**Eat more:**

- Fruit
- Vegetables
- Nuts
- Fish
- Poultry: chicken & turkey

**Eat less:**

- Dairy: cream, milk, cheese, ice cream, butter
- Saturated fat: pork, beef, dairy

**Be moderate:**

- Beer, wine, liquor.

---

Coffee and tea, both green and black, have been shown to be protective against Parkinson's disease. The reason for the benefit is unclear, but theories include the antioxidant content of these beverages, improved bowel habits, and their pleasure-enhancing (and thus dopamine-encouraging) effects.

## Is there a special diet I should eat if I have Parkinson's disease?

No one special diet is recommended for everyone with Parkinsonism. While several studies have identified foods that are associated with an increased, or decreased, risk of Parkinson's disease, not a single study has demonstrated that changing your diet once diagnosed will change the progression of your disease.

There are, however, a few approaches to eating that just make sense if you have Parkinsonism or have a family member who does. It makes sense to avoid foods that are associated with inflammation and disease progression and to eat more of the foods associated with neuroprotection. (See Section entitled: Recommendations for Eating)

# c. HERBAL MEDICINE

Herbal medicines have been used to treat "shaking palsy" for thousands of years. The richest source of herbal therapies to control tremor come from India, where a form of medicine called Ayurveda is commonly practiced.

| Pharmaceutical Medicine | Herbal Medicine |
|---|---|
| STRENGTHS | WEAKNESSES |
| <ul><li>Exact dosage of desired product with each pill.</li><li>Covered by insurance.</li><li>Common language in the US—most US doctors understand what you are on, why you are on it, and the contraindications and side effects.</li></ul> | <ul><li>Inconsistent doses of desired products based on dozens of factors (soil it was grown in, when/ how harvested, etc.)</li><li>Risk of contamination—some of the most notable cases of lead toxicity in recent years have come from contaminated herbal therapies from China and India.</li><li>Most US physicians are unfamiliar with the use, contraindications, and side effects.</li></ul> |

| Pharmaceutical Medicine | Herbal Medicine |
|---|---|
| WEAKNESSES | STRENGTHS |
| • The targeted approach often neglects supporting processes.<br>• Frequent side effects. | • There is a synergy between the ingredients within the plant, that can lead to increased efficacy.<br>• Therapies are often more gentle and cause fewer side effects (not always). |

Herbal medicines come with inherent strengths and weaknesses compared to pharmaceutical medicines.

DO NOT USE IF YOU HAVE PARKINSON'S DISEASE:

### Kava kava, Piper methysticum

Kava kava has been reported to increase the symptoms of Parkinson's disease. The authors of one study concluded that there is competition between dopamine and kava kava that could account for the increase in symptoms.[10]

# d. Art Therapy

By Jessie Lyle

Art Therapy employs the creative process as a means of feeling increased well-being through relaxation and meditative art making. Art Therapy also holds the potential for deepened awareness and insight into internal emotional and cognitive states.

As an Art Therapist living with early onset Parkinson's disease, I have found personally profound results with pain reduction and stopping tremor.

I entered the profession of Art Therapy with a 25-year history of painting, exhibiting, and selling my art. At the start of my art therapy career I worked with clients who were severely debilitated by PD and so began to learn the many faces of PD and what worked when it came to employing the creative process. When I experienced my own first strong PD symptoms, I did not at first understand what was happening. I developed a very stress-responsive tremor. Struggling one month to complete a solo art exhibit while also working full time at a skilled nursing home, I found my fatigue and tremor interfering with my ability to paint and work. Out of the necessity of a deadline, I found when I lay down in bed in a nest of pillows and began to paint, the tremor would quickly stop and allow me to focus and work for hours on detailed, time-intensive images. Before the exhibit came down, I had been diagnosed with Parkinson's, and I immediately began to personally apply what I had learned from my own circumstance to work with my clients. My first experience of talking a client through her fear that she could not paint to the moment when she took the brush and the tremor subsided, allowing her an hour and a half of playful art making, has moved and inspired me to follow a twofold path of discovery. I have discovered firsthand both how art making can benefit my own daily life with PD and how I can bring that knowledge to the benefit of others living with PD.

*Jessie Lyle is an artist and art therapist living and working in Winthrop, WA. She is a life-long painter with an art therapy specialty in geriatrics and dementia. Jessie works with individuals living with chronic or life threatening illness.*

### Benefits of Art Therapy

| Physical Benefits | Emotional Benefits | Cognitive Benefits |
| --- | --- | --- |
| • Maintain fine motor skills | • Sense of control | • Stimulates cognition |
| • Reduce pain | • Empowering | • An assessment tool for cognitive decline |
| • Stops the tremor temporarily | • Decreases anxiety, fear, and depression | |
| | • Helps one cope with living with the unknown | • Supports creative problem-solving abilities |

# V. 27 Relevant Topics

## Alpha-Lipoic Acid

α-lipoic acid is a fat-soluble antioxidant that has been shown to be beneficial in neurological diseases. It's an important part of cell membranes. It is classified as an 'accessory nutrient'—required for function, like a vitamin, but unlike a vitamin, the body can produce it.

## *How do I know if I have enough α-lipoic acid?*

It is likely that different individuals have different requirements for α-lipoic acid (biochemical individuality). It is a potent antioxidant, and it stands to reason that a brain with excessive production of free radicals (as is seen in PD) would benefit from additional α-lipoic acid supplementation.

## *Have studies been done on α-lipoic acid in Parkinsonism?*

In vitro studies suggest that α-lipoic acid increases the growth and development of new mitochondria. It is well known that a loss of mitochondria contributes to cell death in PD; α-lipoic acid may offer some protection against this process.

## DOC BOX

Using a cell model of PD, 4-week pretreatment of lipoic acid and/or acetyl-L-carnitine (ALC) protected the cells against mitochondrial dysfunction, oxidative damage, and accumulation of alpha-synuclein and ubiquitin. Most notably, this study found that when these nutrients were combined, they worked at 100-1000x lower concentrations than they did individually. They also found that pretreatment with the combined agents increased mitochondrial biogenesis. The study concludes,

> This study provides important evidence that combining mitochondrial antioxidant/nutrients at optimal doses might be an effective and safe prevention strategy for PD.[11]

➤ Suppose α-lipoic acid does increase mitochondrial formation. It would seem a great thing to give to a developing brain (children) or to one deficient in mitochondria (PD patients).

In a model of PD, rats were treated with reserpine (causes PD-like symptoms) with or without lipoic acid. The administration of lipoic acid improved the antioxidant status of the brain, and the authors conclude:

> The mode of [lipoic acid] action ... strongly suggests that this compound may be of therapeutic value in the treatment of Parkinson's disease.[12]

Treatment of fat cells with the combination of lipoic acid and acetyl L-carnitine significantly increased mitochondrial mass, expression of mitochondrial DNA, mitochondrial complexes, oxygen consumption and fatty acid oxidation. The authors conclude that the combination of these two nutrients may act to promote mitochondrial synthesis and adipocyte metabolism.[13]

## DOC BOX

Researchers at the University of California, Irvine have identified a group of nutrients that can directly or indirectly protect mitochondria from oxidative damage and improve mitochondrial function. They have named them "mitochondrial nutrients." They suggest that the administration of mitochondrial nutrients may be an effective strategy to improve mitochondrial and cognitive dysfunction for patients suffering from neurodegenerative diseases.

Direct protection of mitochondria:
- Prevents the generation of oxidants
- Scavenges free radicals
- Inhibits oxidant reactivity
- Elevates cofactors of defective mitochondrial enzymes with increase Michaelis-Menten constant to stimulate enzyme activity

Indirect protection of mitochondria:
- Repairs oxidative damage by enhancing antioxidant defense systems via
- Activates of phase 2 enzymes
- Increases mitochondrial biogenesis.[14]

# What is the suggested dose of alpha lipoic acid?

Alpha lipoic acid has not been studied in individuals with Parkinson's disease. For other diseases, such as peripheral neuropathy and diabetes, doses between 600-1200mg are generally used.

# Aluminum

Aluminum is a well-known neurotoxin that accumulates in the substantia nigra of individuals affected by Parkinson's disease.[15]

## *Does aluminum exposure cause or contribute to PD?*

Nobody knows what causes PD exactly, but many studies have implicated environmental factors, especially pesticides and metals, as contributing factors. (See Section entitled: Pesticides) On a cellular level, one of the earliest abnormalities is the formation of "gunk" within neurons, more properly referred to as a-synuclein and fibrils. It is well-known that exposure to pesticides will lead to the formation of this gunk within the brain; what is newly established is that the presence of metals, especially aluminum, will drastically accelerate this process.[16]

No study has specifically looked at exposure to aluminum and the risk of PD. One study did look at the risk of developing Alzheimer's disease, a related neurodegenerative disorder, and the use of aluminum-containing products. The researchers concluded that the use of aluminum-containing deodorant was associated with a greater incidence of Alzheimer's disease.[17]

## *What are the primary sources of aluminum exposure?*

The main source of aluminum intake is food, where it is used as an additive in processed cheese, baked goods, and grain products, and where it is used as a preservative, coloring agent, and leavening agent. Aluminum occurs in some drinking water naturally, and many water treatment facilities add aluminum in water processing. Antiperspirants, antacids, and vaccines are notable routes of exposure.[18]

Ammonium alum is used in water purification and sewage treatment and as a food additive.

➜ Filter your water

Aluminum chlorohydrate is used in over-the-counter anti-perspirants.

➜ Use deodorant, not aluminum-containing antiperspirants.

➜ Eat organically grown food.

Aluminum hydroxide is used as an antacid and in water purification.

➜ Do not use aluminum-containing antacids or baking powder.

Aluminum phosphate is used in cosmetics.

➜ Only use aluminum-free cosmetics.

## How can I reduce my exposure to aluminum?

➜ Don't drink from aluminum cans and limit use of aluminum foil.

➜ Filter your water. Ammonium alum is used in water purification and sewage treatment.

➔ Use deodorant, not anti-perspirant. Aluminum chlorohydrate is used in over-the-counter anti-perspirants.

➔ Eat organically grown foods. Aluminum phophide is a registered pesticide and insecticide.

➔ Avoid aluminum-containing antacids or baking powder.

➔ Use aluminum-free cosmetics. Aluminum phosphate is used in cosmetics.

➔ Request preservative-free vaccines and limit exposure to unnecessary vaccinations. Aluminum salts are added to many vaccines, to boost the immune response.

# Antioxidants

Oxidative damage is highly involved in the pathogenesis of PD. Antioxidants/nutrients capable of attenuating oxidative damage have been suggested as a treatment strategy in PD.

Antioxidants represent a large class of compounds, defined by their ability quiet free radicals. Several studies have been done inquiring whether antioxidants can affect the course of PD. Unfortunately, most of these studies were done while our understanding of antioxidant chemistry was in its infancy.

## Why are antioxidants studied in Parkinsonism?

The tissue destruction of PD is, in large part, caused by free radicals. Antioxidants offset the damage of free radicals. How to replace them, the right doses, and forms, is not yet understood.

## Why have previous antioxidant studies been unsuccessful?

**Antioxidants are not all the same.** The cleanest way to do a study is to have all variables be the same, except the single agent being studied. That way, we know without question that it is the agent in question imparting the change. This is how antioxidants have been studied in PD. Different doses of vitamin E, or vitamin C, have been given to individuals with PD, and researchers measure to see if the antioxidant affected the disease. Most often, it has not.

"Antioxidant" refers to an entire class of molecules that is defined

47

by its activity—to quench free radicals. By their nature, antioxidants are constantly being recycled. They never work alone—their activity depends on interactions with free radicals and other antioxidants.

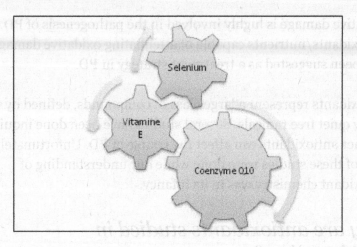

**Research favors single-agent studies, but antioxidants are a part of a complex.** Antioxidants work as part of a complex system. They can only be understood with respect to surrounding tissue, contents, and processes. PD researchers are leading the way towards a paradigm shift—recent publications suggest looking at a system-wide approach.

Progressive thinkers in medicine have suggested Parkinsonism stands to benefit tremendously from a whole-systems approach. Topics for future research include:

- Targeting cellular energy production in neurological disorders.[19]

- Bioenergetic approaches for neuroprotection in Parkinson's disease.[20]

- Neurodegeneration from mitochondrial insufficiency: nutrients, stem cells, growth factors, and prospects for brain rebuilding using integrative management.[21]

- Cellular stress response: a novel target for chemoprevention and nutritional neuroprotection in aging, neurodegenerative disorders and longevity.[22]

## What causes excessive ROS/free radical production in brains with PD?

What comes first, the chicken or the egg? Nobody is sure whether the free radical excess is caused by an increased production of free radicals, or an antioxidant system unable to keep up.

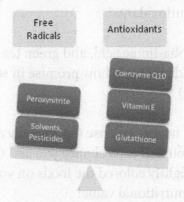

Healthy brains are constantly producing free radicals. Antioxidants produced by the body (endogenous) and dietary antioxidants (exogenous) work together to keep the free radical burden in check. Is the problem the excessive production of free radicals, or an insufficient ability to manage them?

Regardless, a reasonable strategy is:

- Discourage the production of free radicals

- Encourage the availability of antioxidants

**Make the brain healthier!**

# Which antioxidants show promise in PD?

The earlier in the disease that change is implemented, the greater the significance of the change. As was already stated, the late presentation of symptoms in PD makes it very difficult to study prevention. Studies do show that diets high in fruits, vegetables, and especially beans are protective in Parkinsonism.

→ Eat diets rich in fruits, vegetables, and legumes. All are rich sources of antioxidants!

Coenzyme Q-10, alpha-lipoic acid, and green tea polyphenols are examples of antioxidants that show promise in studies. (See individual chapters)

→ Incorporate nutrient-dense (specifically antioxidant-rich) foods into yourself each chance you get! Generally speaking, the more brightly colored the foods on your plate, the greater the nutritional value!

## ORAC (Antioxidant) Content of Various Foods

| | |
|---|---|
| Pinto beans (1/2 cup) | 11864 |
| Red kidney beans (1/2 c) | 13259 |
| Small red beans (1/2 cup) | 13727 |
| Artichoke hearts (1 cup) | 7900 |
| Pecans (1 oz) | 5095 |
| Hazelnuts (1 oz) | 2739 |
| Walnuts (1 oz) | 3846 |
| Popcorn (1 cup) | 157 |
| Whole grain bread (1 slice) | 398 |
| Blueberry (1 cup) | 10000 |
| Blackberry (1 cup) | 7701 |
| Cranberry (1 cup) | 8983 |
| Raspberry (1 cup) | 6058 |
| Strawberry (1 cup) | 5938 |
| Cinnamon (1 gram) | 2675 |
| Turmeric (1 gram) | 1592 |
| Cloves (1 gram) | 3144 |
| Oregano, dried (1g) | 2001 |
| Ketchup (1 gram) | 6 |

An increased production of free radicals is a known contributor to the Parkinson's disease process. Antioxidants quell free radicals, like water on a fire. Antioxidants are abundant in brightly colored fruits and vegetables, spices, and beans. Given that the side effects of increasing antioxidants in your diet is better overall health, decreased risk of cancer, heart disease, and dementia ... why not?

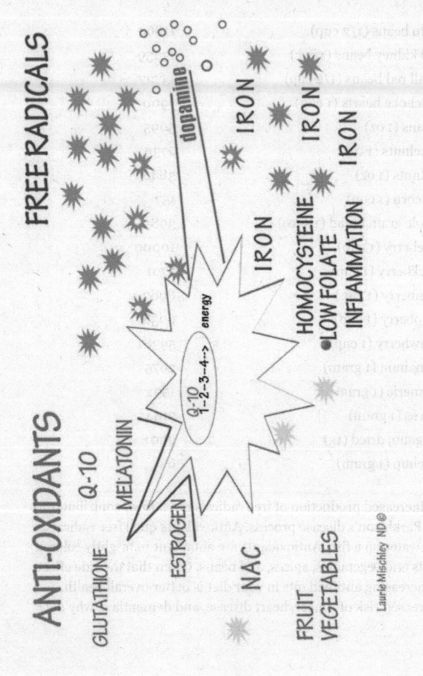

FREE RADICALS

ANTI-OXIDANTS

Q-10

GLUTATHIONE    MELATONIN

ESTROGEN

NAC

FRUIT
VEGETABLES

Q-10
1–2–3–4–› energy

dopamine

IRON    IRON    IRON    IRON

IRON

HOMOCYSTEINE
●LOW FOLATE
INFLAMMATION

Laurie Mischley ND©

# Beta-carotene

Carotenoids are naturally occurring pigments from the chloroplasts and chromoplasts of plants and small organisms. There are over 600 known carotentoids, many of which have been shown to act as antioxidants. Carotene gives apricots and carrots their bright orange color.

## Have carotenoids been studied in Parkinson's disease?

Beta-carotene has been shown to prevent and break up the accumulation of protein aggregates found in Parkinson's disease, Lewy Body disease, and multiple system atrophy. The authors concluded:

> With such potent anti-fibrillogenic as well as fibril-destabilizing activities, these compounds could be useful in the treatment and prevention of Lewy body diseases and multiple system atrophy.[23]

---

### DOC BOX

Vitamin A, beta-carotene, and coenzyme Q10 dose-dependently inhibited the formation of alpha-synuclein fibrils. Moreover, they also dose-dependently destabilized preformed fibrils.[24]

---

## How can I get more beta-carotene?

Beta carotene is the orange pigment common in many fruits and vegetables. Examples are yellow and red bell peppers, carrots, carrot juice, orange zucchini, and apricots.

Eat food rich in carotenoids! See how many shades of red and yellow you can add to your diet.

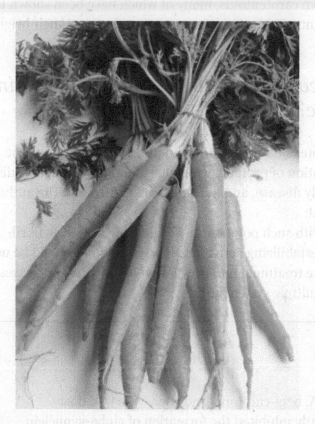

## *Is there anything I can do to increase the absorption of carotenoids?*

One study showed that the addition of avocado fruit and oil significantly enhanced the absorption of all four carotenoids tested.[25]

Oils are an essential part of a healthy diet, especially those coming from plants. When cooking and making salads, be liberal with your use of olive, avocado, sunflower oil, safflower, and canola oils. Try adding nuts and nut butters to vegetable dishes: i.e. squash and cashew casserole.

It's fascinating that foods high in carotenoids contain very little fat. And yet fat make them work better in the body. Diverse foods with different nutritional properties must be eaten in various combinations to cover our nutritional bases. This is a perfect example of the complexity of nutrition.

**RECIPE**: Stuffed orange zucchini. Scrape out the contents of the squash with a spoon, sauté with oil garlic, onions, spices. Refill and bake.

# Calorie Restriction

Overeating is a major modifiable risk factor for several age-related diseases, including Parkinson's disease, Alzheimer's disease, cardiovascular disease, and diabetes.[26] Calorie restriction is usually defined as 10-25% less caloric intake than the average Western diet.

## How much food should somebody eat?

Humans throughout history, and majority of people on the planet now, are having a hard time obtaining food. The amount of food one should eat has only recently become a subject of study. Weight should be relatively stable, neither under or overweight.

## Will I lose weight?

Researchers at the Washington University School of Medicine in St. Louis studied the effects of a calorie restricted diet for 10-25% less caloric intake than the average Western diet. BMI 25.9 in controls, 19.6 in CR group. Nearly all the decreases in BMI occurred in the first year of dieting.

## How much food is too much?

If your belly is bigger than your hips, you're probably eating too much, and the wrong things, too. A high waist-to-hip ratio is one of the leading predictors of cardiovascular disease and diabetes. (Interestingly, all of these conditions, and also PD, have been shown to benefit from nutrient-dense foods, fiber, and omega-3 oils.)

# DOC BOX

## Dietary Restriction is Neuroprotective

In a rodent model of PD, a calorie restriction (CR) diet (30% reduced) decreased the progression of PD. Animals that had been fed the reduced-intake diet had more dopamine in their brains, and more glial-cell-line-derived neurotrophic factor (GDNF), a small protein that potently promotes the survival of many types of neurons. GDNF's most prominent feature is its ability to support the survival of dopaminergic and motorneurons.[27]

## Dietary Restriction Stimulates Neural Stem Cells in the Brain to Produce New Nerve Cells

"Dietary restriction increased the production of brain-derived neurotrophic factor (BDNF), which can enhance learning and memory, can protect neurons against oxidative and metabolic insults, and can stimulate neurogenesis, all actions that may protect neurons against age-related neurodegenerative disorders." "Therefore, it appears that dietary restriction promotes neuronal survival, plasticity, and even neurogenesis by inducting a mild cellular stress response that involves activation of genes that encode proteins designed to promote neuronal growth and survival."[28]

Food restriction reduces brain damage and improves behavioral outcome following excitotoxic and metabolic insults:

Food restriction (FR) in rodents is known to extend life span, reduce the incidence of age-related tumors, and suppress oxidative damage to proteins, lipids, and DNA in several organ systems. Excitotoxicity and mitochondrial impairment are believed to play major roles in the neuronal degeneration and death that occurs in the brains of patients suffering from both acute brain insults such as stroke and seizures, and chronic neurodegenerative conditions such as Alzheimer's, Parkinson's, and Huntington's diseases ... These findings suggest that FR not only extends life span, but increases resistance of the brain to insults that involve metabolic compromise and excitotoxicity.[29]

## What about weight loss and nutritional deficiency?

There are very real and concerning risks of "calorie restriction diets," and this is the major reason such diets are rarely recommended. **Choosing foods is a game of strategy. Don't each too much, and make what you do eat count.**

## What if I'm already underweight?

Being underweight comes with different risk factors. BMI should always be at least 19. It is not healthy to be underweight!

Individuals with PD are already at increased risk of malnutrition. Medications often interfere with nutrients (i.e. protein, folic acid), mobility is an issue (food prep carries additional burden), and individuals with PD are more likely to be constipated and secondarily reduce intake.

## Choosing Nutrient—Dense Foods

Nutrient dense foods are exactly how they sound—foods that don't take up unnecessary space in your gut, foods whose caloric content is rich in vitamins, minerals, healthy fats, and accessory nutrients. Foods such as bread, pasta, pastries, chips, fries, and dairy provide a disproportionate amount of calories with very little nutritional value. See if you can comprise your diet from the following foods:

### NUTRIENT-DENSE FOODS

**A**rtichokes, Apricots, Apples, Amaranth, Arugula, Avocado

**B**ananas, Beans, Berries, Broccoli, Beets, Bok choy, Brussels sprouts

**C**urry, Collards, Coconut, Capers, Cabbage, Chard, Cucumbers

**D**uck, Daikon, Dandelion greens

**E**ggplant, Endive

**F**ish, Figs

**G**ourds, Garbanzo beans, Garlic, Green beans

**H**erring, Hummus, Halibut

**I**ndian curry, Iced tea, Italian dressing

**J**ambalaya, Juice,

**K**ale, Kohlrabi, Kidney beans, Kiwi, Kumquat

**L**egumes, Lettuce, Leeks, Liver

**M**elons, Mushrooms, Miso

**N**uts, Nectarines

**O**ranges, Oats, Okra, Olives, Onions

**P**omegranate, Pickles, Peas, Parsnips, Plums, Peaches

**Q**uiche, Quail

**R**ice, Radish, Rhubarb

**S**pinach, Squash, Strawberries

**T**urnips, Turmeric, Tomatoes, Turkey, Tahini

**U**gli fruit
**V**enison, Vindaloo,
**W**atercress, Watermelon, Waldorf salad, wild rice
**X**igua
**Y**am, Yolks, Yellow squash, Yucca
**Z**ucchini

**Ugli** fruit
**Venison**, Vindaloo,
**Watercress**, Watermelon, Waldorf salad, wild rice
**Xigua**
**Yam**, Yolks, Yellow squash, Yucca
**Zucchini**

# Carnitine

Carnitine is derived from the amino acid, lysine. Under certain conditions, the demand for L-carnitine may exceed an individual's capacity to synthesize it, making it a conditionally essential micronutrient.[30] Parkinson's disease is likely one of those conditions.

## *Why is carnitine being studied in Parkinson's disease?*

L-carnitine plays an important role in reducing the brain injury associated with mitochondrial neurodegenerative disorders.

## *Where does carnitine come from?*

Our bodies make some, and the rest comes from diet. Heart and skeletal muscle contain the greatest concentrations of carnitine, and thus vegetarians are at an increased risk of deficiency.

> → If you don't eat meat, you should take a carnitine supplement.

## *How much carnitine do I need?*

The amount you need from diet depends on your body's demand for carnitine and your ability to supply that demand internally. That which cannot be supplied should be eaten as food or otherwise supplemented.

## DOC BOX

Using a cell model of PD, 4-week pretreatment of lipoic acid and/or acetyl-L-carnitine (ALC) protected the cells against mitochondrial dysfunction, oxidative damage, and accumulation of alpha-synuclein and ubiquitin. Most notably, this study found that when these nutrients were combined, they worked at 100 to 1000 fold lower concentrations than they did individually. The researchers also found that pretreatment with the combined agents **increased mitochondrial biogenesis.** The study concludes, "This study provides important evidence that combining mitochondrial antioxidant/nutrients at optimal doses might be an effective and safe prevention strategy for PD."[31]

# Chelation

Chelation is the act of removing metals from the body. There are many different metals that one might want to remove from the body, and there are at least as many chelating agents.

## Should I undergo chelation if I have Parkinsonism?

Chelation has not been studied in PD. You should absolutely not chelate yourself, or work with a provider offering to chelate you, if you do not know—specifically—what you are trying to get out. For each metal, there are preferable chelating agents. Each chelating agent comes with its own risks, side effects, and efficacy profile.

## What if I am told I have heavy metal toxicity?

If you are told you have heavy metal toxicity, this should be taken very seriously. Unfortunately, the term "toxicity" means different things to different people. On what is this assessment based? Get copies of all relevant labs and take them to at least one other practitioner for a second opinion.

## If I do have lab results suggestive of lead, copper, aluminum, or manganese excess, what should I do?

You should consult a physician trained in environmental medicine, and preferably neurology. Each one of the above metals is treated differently, and most of them are not managed with chelation.

## What are the risks of chelation?

As already stated, chelation has not been studied in Parkinsonism. The most significant risk is that "stirring up the pot" will re-expose the body. Presumably, the body didn't have the means or resources to eliminate the toxicant during first exposure. And the chelating agents themselves each come with risks—to the kidney, liver, and electrolyte status of the individual.

**Don't even consider chelation unless you:**

- Know what metal you're trying to eliminate.

- Know where the source of exposure was. (Make sure you're not still being exposed.)

- Have healthy, functioning processes of elimination: kidney health, liver health, daily bowel movement, frequent water consumption and urination.

- Exercise and sweat regularly.

# Cholesterol

High total and LDL cholesterol are correlated with increased risk of atherosclerosis and cardiovascular disease. Because of this association, cholesterol has gotten a reputation as being "bad" in recent years.

Contrary to popular belief, cholesterol is one of the most valuable nutrients for our body. With it, we make cell membranes, sex hormones, vitamin D, and dozens of other molecules. It is important to maintain optimal levels of cholesterol in your body. Cholesterol should neither be too high nor too low.

## What is the optimal range for cholesterol?

Blood levels should be between 175-200 mg/dL.

## Is my cholesterol too low?

Optimal cholesterol levels are between 180-200mg/dL. 160-220mg/dL are acceptable. If your total cholesterol level is below 160mg/dL, you have "cholesterol deficiency." Cholesterol levels below 160mg/dL have been associated with depression, anxiety, and other diseases.

## Why is cholesterol important?

Cholesterol is essential for the normal function of the body. All mammalian cells require cholesterol for cell membrane permeability and fluidity. It serves as the basic building block for all steroid molecules: testosterone, estrogen, progesterone, DHEA, cortisol, cortisone, aldosterone, and vitamin D, to name a few. It also plays a role in cell signaling, the communication between neurons. Serum cholesterol is the most important determinant of serum levels of coenzyme Q10, a powerful antioxidant.[32]

Cholesterol is especially important in the brain, the most cholesterol-rich organ in the human body. Cholesterol is a major component of neuronal cell membranes and synapses and essential for maintaining their structure and function.[33]

## Is low cholesterol associated with PD?

Lower serum levels of total cholesterol have been described in patients with PD compared with controls.[34,35]

The Rotterdam study, a prospective study conducted over 10 years, concluded that in women, higher levels of serum total cholesterol are associated with significantly decreased risk of developing PD.[36]

One explanation proposed for the link between low cholesterol and PD is the resulting reduction in the production of Q10.[37] (See Section entitled: Coenzyme Q10)

## Where does cholesterol deficiency come from?

Cholesterol is a semi-essential fat; the dietary requirement depends on what your body is able to produce. Some people need to get it from diet, while others can produce plenty in their liver. Cholesterol only comes from animals, so vegans are at increased risk of cholesterol deficiency.

It is routine practice for some doctors to prescribe lipid-lowering agents for anyone with a cholesterol level above 220, or lower. Very few people seem concerned with cholesterol deficiency, defined here as levels below 160.

To ensure adequate levels of cholesterol, blood levels should be checked annually, and the target goal should be 175-200mg/dL. Cholesterol deficiency is defined here as levels below 160mg/dL. Cholesterol excess means levels above 200.

→ If your levels are below 160: Eat more egg yolks, liver, and squid (calamari).

→ If your levels are above 200: Increase your intake of fiber, omega-3 fats, and plant sterols. Increase your physical activity level.

→ If possible, avoid the use of statins as cholesterol lowering agents. They cause a depletion of coenzyme Q10, an especially important nutrient in Parkinsonism. (See Section entitled: Coenzyme Q10)

## What if I'm on a statin to lower my cholesterol?

Statins are a class of pharmaceutical drugs commonly prescribed in the US to lower cholesterol. Dozens of these pharmaceutical drugs exist: some popular examples of statin drugs include atorvastatin (Lipitor), lovastatin (Mevacor), simvistatin (Zocor), simvastatin+ezetimibe (Vytorin), among many others. If you are unsure whether you are on a statin, ask your doctor.

Statins act by interfering with the enzyme in the liver that makes cholesterol, HMG-CoA reductase, the same enzyme needed to produce coenzyme Q10! (See Section entitled: Coenzyme Q10)

# Dietary Sources of Cholesterol

| Food | Serving | Cholesterol (mg) |
|---|---|---|
| Chicken, giblets, cooked, simmered | 1 cup | 641 |
| Turkey, giblets, cooked, simmered | 1 cup | 419 |
| Beef, liver, cooked, pan-fried | 3 oz | 324 |
| Egg, whole, cooked, scrambled | 1 large | 215 |
| Crustaceans, shrimp, canned | 3 oz | 214 |
| Duck, domesticated, meat only, cooked, roasted | ½ duck | 197 |
| Turkey, neck meat only, cooked, simmered | 1 neck | 185 |
| Fish, salmon, sockeye, cooked, dry heat | ½ fillet | 135 |
| Fish, sardine, Atlantic, canned in oil, with bone | 3 oz | 121 |
| Chicken, stewing, meat only, cooked, stewed | 1 cup | 116 |
| Fish, haddock, cooked, dry heat | 1 fillet | 111 |
| Turkey, meat only, cooked, roasted | 1 cup | 106 |
| Crab, blue, crab cakes | 1 cake | 90 |
| Turkey, light meat, cooked, roasted | 1 cup | 58 |
| Salami, cooked, beef and pork | 2 slices | 50 |
| Fish, halibut, Atlantic & Pacific, cooked, dry heat | 3 oz | 35 |
| Fish, ocean perch, Atlantic, cooked, dry heat | 1 fillet | 27 |
| Pork sausage, fresh, cooked | 1 patty | 23 |
| Pork sausage, fresh, cooked | 2 links | 22 |
| Fish, herring, Atlantic, pickled | 3 oz | 11 |
| Foods from plants | 0 | 0 |

If you are on a statin and have Parkinson's disease:

- Revisit the topic of cholesterol management with your doctor. If your doctor is not an expert in preventative medicine, find a naturopathic doctor or nutritionist who can provide counsel on lowering cholesterol with diet and exercise.

- Ensure that you are not being over-medicated. Your cholesterol levels should always be between 175-200 mg/dl.

- Since statins deplete coenzyme Q10, one of the most important nutrients in PD, you must supplement with at least 100mg/day coenzyme Q10.

# Choline

Choline is an essential nutrient, required for cell membranes and the production of the brain neurotransmitter, acetylcholine. Acetylcholine is most well known for its role in learning and memory.

## Can I get choline from my diet?

Choline is usually delivered from food in the form phosphatidylcholine. The richest sources in the diet include egg yolks, soy, wheat germ, and liver. You'll notice that most chocolate bars contain soy lecithin: lecithin is the emulsifier that prevents the cocoa and cocoa butter from separating!

## Can I take a choline supplement?

The most widely available forms of choline supplements are lecithin and phosphatidylcholine, which are usually derived from egg yolks or soy. Lecithin is usually sold in a container of granules—some people add them to their morning oatmeal. Phosphatidylcholine is usually sold in pill form.

## What does choline have to do with Parkinson's?

Choline is being studied as a nutrient for brain health. Preliminary studies suggest that it plays a role in neuroprotection and neurorepair. While there was some very promising research done on choline and Parkinson's in the 80's, there has been very little follow-up since.

## Are individuals with PD deficient in choline?

Very few studies have been done looking at the nutrient requirements specific to PD. One study demonstrated that individuals with Parkinson's disease have less choline in their cerebral spinal fluid (CSF), whether or not they were being treated with levodopa (p=0.0001). The authors of this study attributed reduced levels of choline in CSF to a deficit in choline transport into the brain, or a decrease in choline-phospholipid output from the brain.[38]

## Will supplementing with choline help my PD symptoms?

In the late 1980's, researchers in Spain studied the effects of a particular form of choline, cytidine diphosphate choline (CDP-choline, citicoline), in PD. Individuals participating in the study had been on levodopa for several years, and added 500mg/day of CDP-choline for 30 days. At the end of the 30 days, they were able to reduce their dose of levodopa by about 30%, without reducing medication efficacy![39]

CDP-choline, thought to improve the functionality of the dopamine system, was administered to Parkinsonian patients in a double-blind cross-over study. The CDP-choline supplement showed "a 23% improvement in bradykinesia (slowness) and 33% improvement in rigidity."[40]

## Are there side effects to supplementing with choline?

Choline is quite safe and inexpensive. In one study, patients noticed a temporary increase in their dyskinesias, corrected by reducing their dose of levodopa.

## If I take choline, should I take less levodopa?

Two studies have demonstrated improvement when individuals supplemented with a choline supplement, Citicoline, for 30 days, and then reduced their dose of levodopa by 33-50%. You should try to schedule an appointment with your PD provider about 1 month after beginning supplementation to determine whether your medications need to be adjusted. Bring a copy of the references below if you suspect your provider is not familiar with choline supplementation.

Choline is indicated for individuals looking to reduce their dose of levodopa. 85 patients with PD were given 1200mg of citicoline daily. More improvements on the PD tests were shown by those patients who received half their levodopa dose than those who stayed on their usual dose![41]

In a study done in 1988, individuals developed a worsening of dyskinesias while supplementing with CDP-choline. Researchers discovered that participants on their usual dose of levodopa were essentially over-medicated with the addition of choline. After 30 days of supplementation with choline, the dose of levodopa was reduced by one-third, and the incidence of dyskinesia dropped to its previous levels, but the therapeutic response remained stable. A significant increase in the number of lymphocytic dopaminergic receptors also occurred.

## What's the best form of choline to take?

Citicoline, cytidine diphosphate-choline (CDP-Choline), is the form that has been researched the most. It is widely available online by the name Citicoline.

➔ Recommended dose: 500-1200mg/day.

Lecithin usually comes in granules or in a gelcap. Most forms of choline are quite inexpensive.

➔ 1 tbsp lecithin granules on your oatmeal or applesauce each morning.

# Coenzyme Q-10

In 2002, researchers from the University of California, San Diego reported that high doses of coenzyme Q10 were able to slow to progression of PD by almost 40%.[42] This was terribly exciting, given that no other therapies have been shown to curb the course of the disease to this extent. So why isn't everyone taking it?

That study was only trying to answer the question, "is high-dose Q10 safe?" It looked at Q10's effect on disease progression secondarily. For very good and very complicated reasons, researchers can only answer the primary question being asked.

The authors concluded that high dose Q10 was safe and recommended follow-up studies with more people, for longer periods, using higher doses[43] to help determine whether Q10 at this, and possibly higher, dosages truly derails the progression of PD. In this study, lower doses did not slow the progression of the disease substantially.

A follow-up study is currently underway investigating 1200mg, 2400mg, and placebo.

## Why not take high-dose coenzyme Q10?

Given its apparent safety and preliminary research suggesting it may be helpful, you may be asking yourself "Why not?" The cost for high quality coenzyme Q10 (used in the study) is about $200-400/month! Until more research is done, individuals are left to guess whether or not the supplement is slowing their disease or wasting their money.

## How does coenzyme Q10 work?

Q10 probably works via several mechanisms in Parkinson's disease. It functions as an antioxidant but also promotes the health and function of the mitochondria. (Mitochondrial loss is a well-established problem in Parkinsonism.)

## Are all forms of coenzyme Q10 the same?

Until more research is done, we don't know the answer to that question. As with most over-the-counter supplements, quality control standards are lacking. The study with the best results thus far used a wafer form of Q10. In addition to Q10, the wafer included a bit of fat (to improve absorption) and vitamin E, to maintain its antioxidant status.

- Vitaline wafers and Douglas Labs CoQ-melt are examples of high-quality coenzyme Q10 products.

# Constipation

Constipated men are more than 4 times more likely to develop Parkinson's disease than those who have 2 or more bowel movements per day!

## *How do I know if I'm constipated?*

Constipation is defined as less than one bowel movement (BM) per day. Constipation is common among the elderly, and even more common among those with Parkinson's disease. For years this was seen as a result either of the inactivity associated with the disease or of a poorly functioning nervous system.

A better look at the research suggests that individuals who are constipated in midlife are quite a bit more likely to develop PD. Constipated men were 4.1 time more likely to develop PD than men who had 2 BM/day. The risk of developing PD was even lower in men who had more than 2 bowel movements per day.[44]

What about women? We don't know. These findings, the best to date, were based on the Honolulu Heart Study, which only included men. Research on women hasn't been done yet.

Follow-up studies show that there is a correlation between BM frequency and protection against forming incidental Lewy bodies, which are protein aggregates that occur in the brain long before symptoms of PD develop.

## *Why is constipation associated with Parkinson's disease?*

Nobody knows why constipation is associated with an increased risk of developing PD. Current theories include:

- Constipation is an early marker of disease, predating other symptoms by years.

- Reduced elimination of toxicants. The bowels are one of the primary routes of eliminating unwanted waste and dangerous byproducts. When stool sits in the colon, the toxicants are reabsorbed into the bloodstream and recirculated throughout the body.

- Some PD medications increase constipation, making the problem worse.

## Can bowel movements be protective against PD?

On autopsy, individuals who had one or more bowel movements per day had significantly higher density of substantial nigral neurons. Whether or not constipated individuals had Lewy bodies, those who had less than one bowel movement per day had a thinning of the substantia nigra, the part of the brain most severely affected in PD.[45]

## How much water is enough?

As trite as it may seem, insufficient intake of water is one of the most common causes of constipation. This is especially true in Parkinson's disease. One study looking at constipation in PD found that individuals who were most constipated reported never feeling thirsty, in spite of reduced bowel movements.

Even if you're not thirsty, try to increase your water consumption by 2-4 glasses per day and notice how it affects your bowels. Some individuals find that water containing electrolytes, such as mineral water or rehydration formulas, work even better. Teas, juice, and other beverages count as well.

- Be careful, though: too much coffee or alcohol can contribute to dehydration.
- Eat slowly, chew food thoroughly.
- Drink 48-72 oz of water per day—this includes tea and juice.
- Try to eat plenty of easily digestible warm foods—soups, stews, and hot tea. Just as you put ice on an injury to discourage blood flow, cold 'freezes' up gut function. (This is especially important in Chinese medicine.) Imagine warm foods and fluids causing blood flow to rush to the gut, improving digestion.
- Start the day with warm tea (even hot water & lemon juice) and physical activity. Moving our legs and abdominal muscles helps pump blood through the gut, getting things moving.
- Take time for a morning bowel movement, or when you are most relaxed. Don't ignore urges.
- Avoid stress. Most people have heard of the "fight or flight" part of the nervous system, but "rest and digest" part gets less attention. They are equally important. Your intestines work best when you are relaxed.
- Use a footstool in your bathroom for your feet to mimic the 'squatting' position. Our bodies are designed to have a bowel movement in the squatting position, it's how 2/3 of the world's population does it.
- Eat 30-35 grams/day of fiber per day.

Many patients attempt to relieve the constipation that often accompanies Parkinson's by eating bran. But recent research shows that bran is high in vitamin B-6, which interferes with the effectiveness of levodopa when the drug is taken alone. Prune juice, grains, and fiber laxatives should be substituted instead.

Constipation is very common due to the disease and/or to the medications used to treat PD. Chronic constipation can raise the risk for fecal impaction and colon cancer. Therefore, safe methods of controlling constipation are a necessary part of healthy function.

## SOURCES OF FIBER

Legumes (1 cup)

| | |
|---|---|
| Navy beans | 19g |
| Kidney beans | 16g |
| Split peas | 16g |
| Lentils | 15g |
| Refried beans | 13g |

Cereals & Grains (1 cup)

| | |
|---|---|
| 100% wheat bran | 17g |
| Quinoa | 9g |
| Bulgar | 8g |
| Oat bran | 6g |
| Instant oatmeal | 4g |

Vegetables (1 cup)

| | |
|---|---|
| Artichoke hearts | 9g |
| Spinach, frozen | 7g |
| Brussels sprouts | 7g |
| Winter squash | 6g |

Fruits (1 cup)

| | |
|---|---|
| Prunes | 12g |
| Asian pear (1 pear) | 10g |
| Raspberries and Blackberries | 8g |

Nuts & Seeds (1 oz)          2-3g

The typical American eats 11g of fiber per day. Health experts recommend a minimum of 20-30 grams per day for most people.

# Creatine

Creatine is a nitrogen-rich organic acid that plays a role mitochondrial health and energy production.

## Can creatine slow the progression of Parkinson's disease?

One study concluded that 10 grams/day of creatine slowed the progression of Parkinson's in patients with a recent diagnosis (within 5 years). Another study of 60 individuals with PD who took creatine for two years found those taking creatine had improved mood and smaller dose increases of dopaminergic therapy. This study varied the dose between 2 grams/day and 20 grams/day.[46]

The NIH National Institute of Neurological Disorders and Stroke is currently funding a study at the University of Rochester attempting to determine whether 5 grams/day of creatine is able to slow disease progression over the 5 years of the study.[47]

## Are there any side effects to taking creatine?

The most common side effect of creatine is nausea, and this seems to be dose-dependent. Creatine can also cause dehydration, so it is important to consume plenty of water when using the supplement.

The cost for a month supply of creatine is approximately $10.

# Curcumin (Turmeric)

Turmeric, an Indian spice, contains curcumin, which has been shown to prevent the loss of glutathione and acts as an antioxidant. It has a mild taste and can be added to many dishes.

→ Use turmeric liberally! Add it to scrambled eggs, chicken, and vegetables.

## *How does curcumin protect the brain?*

- It contains antioxidant and anti-inflammatory phenolic compounds.[48]

- It inhibits aggregation of Parkinson-related proteins. Curcumin inhibited alpha-synuclein aggregation in a dose-dependent manner and increased alpha-synuclein solubility in an in vitro model.[49]

- It alleviates the effects of glutathione (GSH) depletion In early PD, there is a significant depletion of the antioxidant glutathione. This depletion results in mitochondrial dysfunction, oxidative stress, and ultimately cell death.

Researchers treated mice and dopaminergic neuronal cells with curcumin—curcumin restored the depletion of glutathione levels, protected against protein oxidation, and preserved mitochondrial dysfunction! The researchers conclude, "These data suggest that curcumin has potential therapeutic value for neurodegenerative diseases involving GSH depletion-mediated oxidative stress."[50]

- It acts as a natural metal chelating agent. A study was done on rats exposed to aluminum (See Section entitled:

Aluminum) in their drinking water. When the rats were given 30mg/kg/day of curcumin, there was a reduction in the damage caused by aluminum. The authors conclude:

> Our results indicate that curcumin's ability to bind redox active metals and cross the blood-brain-barrier could be playing a crucial role in preventing against Al-induced neurotoxicity.[51]

# Dairy

Dairy intake is clearly associated with and increased risk of PD.

In research, it is very difficult to answer the question, "Are there certain foods that, when consumed, increase or decrease an individual's risk of developing PD?" When you take a group of people with PD (or any disease) and ask them to think back to what they were eating 10, 20, or 30 years ago, there are plenty of inaccuracies. In research, it is more accurate to take a large population of people, track what they are eating, and watch and see what diseases develop. This type of study is expensive and requires decades of research before the questions are answered. These are called prospective studies.

Three prospective studies have been done in an attempt to answer this question. Interestingly, all three of them identified dairy as a risk factor for developing PD.[52, 53, 54]

## What constitutes dairy?

First, let's make sure everyone knows exactly what a serving of dairy is. The most commonly consumed dairy items in the United States are: **milk, butter, cheese, cream, ½ & ½, ice cream, sour cream, cottage cheese, cream cheese, yogurt, frozen yogurt, and whey protein supplements.** The data suggest that individuals who consume 3-6 servings of dairy per day have 60-80% greater risk of developing PD than those who rarely or never consume it. Men seem to be more vulnerable to the link than women.

# Why the link between dairy and PD?

Theories addressing this connection include:

- The content of fat, the presence of the sugar (lactose), or the protein (a common allergen)

- Dairy may contain a toxicant (tetrahydroisoquinolines)

- Dairy may be contaminated with pesticides or other persistent organic pollutants

## DOC BOX

Tetrahydroisoquinolines are endogenous neurotoxins, known to cause a Parkinsonism-like syndrome in rodents and primates. They can pass easily through the blood-brain barrier, but cannot be metabolized in the brain or the liver. These endogenously produced substances have been hypothesized to be possible Parkinson's disease-inducing substances.

## Alternatives to Common Dairy Foods

- Milk: rice, almond, soy, hemp, and hazelnut milk to name a few.

- Ice cream: Coconut Bliss is made with coconut milk instead of cow milk.

- Cheese: Veganaise and Wildwood Farms Aioli are excellent spreads.

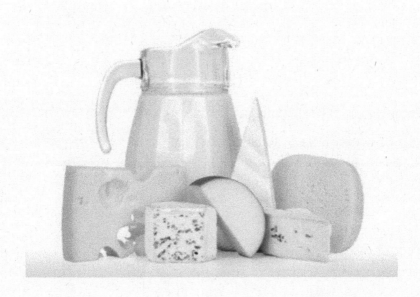

# DHA (fish oil)

"DHA may represent a new approach to improve the quality of life of Parkinson's disease patients."[55]

Fish oil contains a fat, DHA, that plays a role in the survival of dopaminergic neurons. Canadian researchers used a monkey model of Parkinson's disease to study the effects of DHA on PD monkeys taking levodopa.

## Can fish oil reduce dyskinesias?

Dyskinesias are the writhing movements individuals often experience as a result of their medications.

One study concluded that DHA reduced levodopa-induced dyskinesias by about 35% within 4 days of taking the supplement. It is important to note that levodopa retained its ability to reduce Parkinson's symptoms—there were simply fewer side effects. The authors of the study concluded that administration of DHA has the potential to improve quality of life in patients with PD.[56]

## How much fish oil do I need to take to obtain these benefits?

The researchers estimate that the doses used in the study translate to 5-10g DHA/day in humans. Because fish oil is a blend of DHA and other fats, it's difficult to find concentrated forms of DHA.

- Pharmax High DHA Finest Fish Oil is one of the highest quality, most-concentrated, least expensive forms available.

93

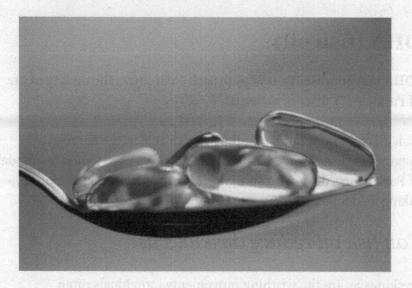

The cost of 7 grams per day ranges from $60 to $210. To get this amount of DHA, one may need to take up to 28 capsules per day!

- High quality liquid is more convenient and often less expensive. It doesn't taste nearly as bad as many people think it might!

## Can I increase DHA in my diet by eating more fish?

The following are some natural sources of DHA: (3 oz)

| | |
|---|---|
| Atlantic Salmon | 0.95g |
| Pacific Herring | 0.75g |
| Pacific Sardines | 0.74g |
| Rainbow Trout | 0.44g |
| White tuna (canned) | 0.54g |
| Light tuna (canned) | 0.19g |

# Fava Beans

Fava beans, also called broad beans, are a natural source of levodopa.

## *Where do fava beans come from?*

Fava beans are native to north Africa and southwest Asia and are cultivated extensively throughout the world. They became part of the eastern Mediterranean diet around 6000 BC.

## *Why the variability of levodopa content in the beans?*

The highest concentration of L-dopa is found in the young beans, especially when consumed with the pod. Approximately ½ cup of fresh green fava beans or 3 oz of canned green fava beans contain about 50-100mg levodopa.

## *How are fava beans eaten?*

Baghali polow, a traditional Persian dish, is a mixture of fava beans, dill weed, and rice. It is traditionally served with lamb, but tastes great with beef, chicken, or fish.

Fava bean salad can be made in minutes by adding canned fava beans to tomatoes, onion, and cucumber tossed with fresh parsley, lemon juice and olive oil.

**You should NOT experiment with Fava beans and Mucuna if:**

- You take a monoamine oxidase inhibitor (MAOI). Examples include selegiline (Eldepryl, Carbex, deprenyl, Zelapar), rasagiline (Azilect), isocarboxazid (Marplan), phenelzine (Nardil), tranylcypromine (Parnate). MAOIs taken in combination with the above legumes can bring about a dangerous and sometimes fatal increase in blood pressure. You must inform your physician if you intend to experiment!

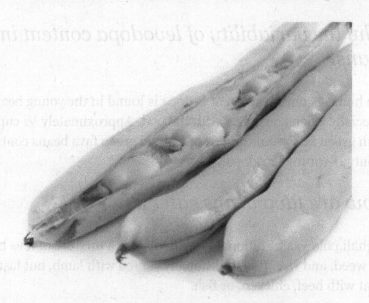

- You have a G6PD deficiency (Favism). Favism is an inherited genetic disease that causes hemolytic anemia, kidney damage, and possibly death upon consumption of fava beans. G6PD deficiency is rare, occurring mostly among people of Mediterranean, African, and Southeast Asian descent, but others can be affected as well. The disorder is usually detected in childhood, but a blood test can be performed to determine if you are at risk.

younger the child when a parent develops Parkinson's disea
greater the risk of Parkinson's disease to that child.[63]

## hat if my infection is very mild? My labs e weakly positive, and I have no GI mptoms.

search suggests that "low-density" infection may be sufficient to ger an autoimmune response. It's not so much the level of the H. ori organisms that is to blame: their presence, even in low levels, set off a cascade of reactions in the immune system. It is most ely the response to H.pylori, not the organisms themselves, that laying a role in Parkinson's disease.[64]

## I eliminate the H. pylori from my gut, will I cured of Parkinson's disease?

search suggests that eradication of H. pylori from the gut does cure the disease but does offer some therapeutic advantage. earchers have demonstrated that gait can improve dramatically owing eradication of H. pylori. One researcher observed of a ient, "The initial gait was tentative, stilted, wooden and doll-like. nsequently, it became relaxed, free-flowing and, finally, rous."

# Glutathione

Gluatathione is the brain's most powerful antioxidant. The loss of glutathione appears to be one of the earliest changes in the brains of individuals with PD. The less glutathione in the brain, the more severe the symptoms of Parkinson's disease and the faster the disease progresses.[57] Replenishing glutathione should be an essential part of treating PD. However, at this time, nobody is sure the best way to do that.

## Does intravenous (IV) glutathione help PD?

One study done in Italy in the mid-1990's on 9 PD patients concluded that 600mg IV glutathione given twice a day for a month reduced PD symptoms by 42%.[58]

Since then, the administration of intravenous glutathione has become popularized by Complementary & Alternative Medicine (CAM) providers around the world. Because of the impracticality of administering an IV twice a day, most providers administer the treatment 3x/week.

There are anecdotal reports that the treatment is capable of improving the symptoms of PD, but no follow-up research has been done.

As you can imagine, going in for an intravenous injection three times a week may be difficult to sustain. This is an invasive therapy that quickly becomes expensive, as insurance doesn't cover experimental therapies

## Why can't glutathione be taken orally?

Oral glutathione is not absorbed into the bloodstream or brain. Some studies show that the supplement N—Acetyl Cysteine (NAC) is capable of increasing glutathione levels in the body, but nobody knows whether the levels in the brain go up, or whether supplementation with this nutrient will affect the course of the disease. 1200mg/day of NAC is a reasonable dose and costs about $15 per month.

## Are there other methods of augmenting brain glutathione levels?

Until more research is done, nobody knows how best to accomplish this.

One study is underway looking at a glutathione nose spray in PD patients. It is theoretically possible that intranasal administration will provide glutathione directly into the brain, where it is needed most. Unlike intravenously-administered glutathione, this antioxidant won't have to compete with the lungs and liver for use and may be able to bypass the blood-brain-barrier entirely. This method of administration may have the advantage of delivering glutathione directly to the brain, where it is needed most.

# H. pylori (Helicobacter pylori)

In 1965, it was first documented that individuals with disease were significantly more likely to have had a p Speculation about a role for infectious agents in Park began in 1979.[60]

## How do I know if I'm infected with

Absolute proof comes from intestinal biopsies. Once made, status can be monitored using the urea breath ELISA value for serum anto-urease-IgG antibody.[61]

## Are there any signs that I may be in

Constipation, diarrhea, and nausea are common GI s associated with Helicobacter infection. It is possible and not have any of these symptoms. In H. pylori inf mitochondrial dysfunction in the enterocytes (gut ce of dopamine in the gut. Diarrhea may signify second overgrowth.[62]

- See Lab Tests: ELISA H pylori antibodies, ur

- Doctor's Data Comprehensive Stool Analysis abnormal bacterial and yeast growth (dysbios intestines.

## How is Helicobacter transmitted?

Most Helicobacter infections are transmitted where contact, as among family members. This fits with the

# Homocysteine

## What is homocysteine?

Homocysteine, measured in the blood, is a normal part of metabolism. But elevated levels are linked to Parkinson's disease, atherosclerosis, vascular disease, Alzheimer's disease, depression, and dementia.

Research suggests that in PD, the longer you've had the disease, the higher your homocysteine level. Treatment with levodopa has been shown to raise homocysteine levels even further. Some studies have shown that elevated homocysteine levels are associated with worsening PD motor symptoms, dyskinesias, and a greater likelihood of cognitive symptoms.[65]

## What is the optimal level of homocysteine?

Ideally, blood levels should be less than 10. Conventional reference ranges usually go up to 15, which I believe is too high.

**How can homocysteine levels be lowered?**

| | |
|---|---|
| Folic acid | 400mcg/day |
| Vitamin B-12 | 1000mcg/day (sublingual is preferred) |
| Vitamin B-6 | 10 mg/day |

This formula, virtually guaranteed to lower homocysteine levels, costs approximately $2.75 per month.

- Take a daily B-vitamin, with food, away from PD medications.

This is a perfect example of integrated medicine. Supplementing with the nutrients listed above, you are able to reduce the risk of co-morbidities associated with PD (such as cardiovascular disease and dementia), take levodopa, and reduce the side effects associated with it. You get the benefits while reducing the side effects and risks!

Long-time users of levodopa-carbidopa have since been found to have increased levels of serum homocysteine,[66,67] implicating vitamins B6, folate, and B12.

# Iron

There are deposits of increased iron in the substantia nigra and iron catalyzes the production of free radicals within neurons. Iron is probably not to blame for causing Parkinsonism, but it is part of the disease process and a significant contributor to progression.

## Who is at risk of excess iron?

Menstruation is a natural form of bloodletting, effectively reducing iron levels. Menstruating women are at significantly less risk of developing PD. As soon as a woman goes through menopause, her risk of developing PD parallels that of men.

## Should I get blood work to assess my iron status?

A propensity to accumulate iron could be devastating to someone with Parkinsonism. At least once, all men and non-menstruating women should check their ferritin level and iron binding studies. Disorders of iron storage are quite prevalent and easily treated, but they often go undiagnosed. If your binding studies come out within normal limits, and ferritin levels are less than 100, you don't have to worry about iron excess.

## Should I avoid dietary iron?

I recommend consuming red meat sparingly. This recommendation is only in part because of the iron, and mostly because of the well-established health and environmental benefits of limiting beef consumption.

In a prospective study, total iron intake was not associated with an increased risk of Parkinson's disease. Interestingly, low vitamin C and high intake of dietary non-heme iron was associated.[68]../../../../Owner/AppData/Local/Temp/Temp1_Natural Therapies for Parkinson's Disease.zip/Natural Therapies for Parkinson's Disease.html - 57 Non-heme iron refers to plant-sourced iron: rich sources include spinach, kale, and molasses. Given how nutrient-dense these foods are, and the protective antioxidants they also contain, in addition to non-heme iron, I do not advise avoiding them.

# Manganese

Manganese is a metal that has been shown to cause Parkinsonism. This natural element is a well-established neurotoxin.

## *What are the most common sources of exposure to manganese?*

Symptoms of toxicity usually occur in workers, such as welders and miners, who have been exposed for extended periods of time. The condition of manganese toxicity is called manganism, or welder's disease. Industrial pollution is becoming a more widely recognized source of elevated manganese levels.

Manganese is a naturally occurring element in well water.

- If you are on a well, be sure to use a high-quality water filter and have your water analyzed annually.

## *How can I test my manganese levels?*

Hair and nail tests accurately assess long-term exposure, providing insight into previous exposures. Urine and blood tests are better methods of assessing and screening for ongoing exposure.

- Doctor's Data provides hair analysis that can inexpensively screen for manganese and many other elements.

## *If my manganese levels are elevated, does it mean I don't have Parkinson's disease?*

You may well have manganism, resulting in very similar symptoms.

This is a complicated conversation to be had with your neurologist. You should immediately take measures to identify the source of your exposure and work with a physician trained in environmental medicine to reduce your levels.

## *I was diagnosed with Parkinson's disease by a very good neurologist. Can I assume he/she tested me for manganese?*

Unfortunately, no. Screening for manganese levels is not part of a routine diagnostic evaluation of Parkinsonism.

# Glutathione

Gluatathione is the brain's most powerful antioxidant. The loss of glutathione appears to be one of the earliest changes in the brains of individuals with PD. The less glutathione in the brain, the more severe the symptoms of Parkinson's disease and the faster the disease progresses.[57] Replenishing glutathione should be an essential part of treating PD. However, at this time, nobody is sure the best way to do that.

## Does intravenous (IV) glutathione help PD?

One study done in Italy in the mid-1990's on 9 PD patients concluded that 600mg IV glutathione given twice a day for a month reduced PD symptoms by 42%.[58]

Since then, the administration of intravenous glutathione has become popularized by Complementary & Alternative Medicine (CAM) providers around the world. Because of the impracticality of administering an IV twice a day, most providers administer the treatment 3x/week.

There are anecdotal reports that the treatment is capable of improving the symptoms of PD, but no follow-up research has been done.

As you can imagine, going in for an intravenous injection three times a week may be difficult to sustain. This is an invasive therapy that quickly becomes expensive, as insurance doesn't cover experimental therapies

## Why can't glutathione be taken orally?

Oral glutathione is not absorbed into the bloodstream or brain. Some studies show that the supplement N—Acetyl Cysteine (NAC) is capable of increasing glutathione levels in the body, but nobody knows whether the levels in the brain go up, or whether supplementation with this nutrient will affect the course of the disease. 1200mg/day of NAC is a reasonable dose and costs about $15 per month.

## Are there other methods of augmenting brain glutathione levels?

Until more research is done, nobody knows how best to accomplish this.

One study is underway looking at a glutathione nose spray in PD patients. It is theoretically possible that intranasal administration will provide glutathione directly into the brain, where it is needed most. Unlike intravenously-administered glutathione, this antioxidant won't have to compete with the lungs and liver for use and may be able to bypass the blood-brain-barrier entirely. This method of administration may have the advantage of delivering glutathione directly to the brain, where it is needed most.

# H. pylori (Helicobacter pylori)

In 1965, it was first documented that individuals with Parkinson's disease were significantly more likely to have had a peptic ulcer.[59] Speculation about a role for infectious agents in Parkinsonism began in 1979.[60]

## How do I know if I'm infected with H.pylori?

Absolute proof comes from intestinal biopsies. Once the diagnosis is made, status can be monitored using the urea breath test and an ELISA value for serum anto-urease-IgG antibody.[61]

## Are there any signs that I may be infected?

Constipation, diarrhea, and nausea are common GI symptoms associated with Helicobacter infection. It is possible to be infected, and not have any of these symptoms. In H. pylori infection, there is mitochondrial dysfunction in the enterocytes (gut cells) and a loss of dopamine in the gut. Diarrhea may signify secondary bacterial overgrowth.[62]

- See Lab Tests: ELISA H pylori antibodies, urea breath test

- Doctor's Data Comprehensive Stool Analysis will test for abnormal bacterial and yeast growth (dysbiosis) in your intestines.

## How is Helicobacter transmitted?

Most Helicobacter infections are transmitted where there is close contact, as among family members. This fits with the findings that

101

the younger the child when a parent develops Parkinson's disease, the greater the risk of Parkinson's disease to that child.[63]

## What if my infection is very mild? My labs are weakly positive, and I have no GI symptoms.

Research suggests that "low-density" infection may be sufficient to trigger an autoimmune response. It's not so much the level of the H. pylori organisms that is to blame: their presence, even in low levels, can set off a cascade of reactions in the immune system. It is most likely the response to H.pylori, not the organisms themselves, that is playing a role in Parkinson's disease.[64]

## If I eliminate the H. pylori from my gut, will I be cured of Parkinson's disease?

Research suggests that eradication of H. pylori from the gut does not cure the disease but does offer some therapeutic advantage. Researchers have demonstrated that gait can improve dramatically following eradication of H. pylori. One researcher observed of a patient, "The initial gait was tentative, stilted, wooden and doll-like. Subsequently, it became relaxed, free-flowing and, finally, vigorous."

# Homocysteine

## *What is homocysteine?*

Homocysteine, measured in the blood, is a normal part of metabolism. But elevated levels are linked to Parkinson's disease, atherosclerosis, vascular disease, Alzheimer's disease, depression, and dementia.

Research suggests that in PD, the longer you've had the disease, the higher your homocysteine level. Treatment with levodopa has been shown to raise homocysteine levels even further. Some studies have shown that elevated homocysteine levels are associated with worsening PD motor symptoms, dyskinesias, and a greater likelihood of cognitive symptoms.[65]

## *What is the optimal level of homocysteine?*

Ideally, blood levels should be less than 10. Conventional reference ranges usually go up to 15, which I believe is too high.

**How can homocysteine levels be lowered?**

| | |
|---|---|
| Folic acid | 400mcg/day |
| Vitamin B-12 | 1000mcg/day (sublingual is preferred) |
| Vitamin B-6 | 10 mg/day |

This formula, virtually guaranteed to lower homocysteine levels, costs approximately $2.75 per month.

- Take a daily B-vitamin, with food, away from PD medications.

This is a perfect example of integrated medicine. Supplementing with the nutrients listed above, you are able to reduce the risk of co-morbidities associated with PD (such as cardiovascular disease and dementia), take levodopa, and reduce the side effects associated with it. You get the benefits while reducing the side effects and risks!

Long-time users of levodopa-carbidopa have since been found to have increased levels of serum homocysteine,[66,67] implicating vitamins B6, folate, and B12.

# Iron

There are deposits of increased iron in the substantia nigra and iron catalyzes the production of free radicals within neurons. Iron is probably not to blame for causing Parkinsonism, but it is part of the disease process and a significant contributor to progression.

## Who is at risk of excess iron?

Menstruation is a natural form of bloodletting, effectively reducing iron levels. Menstruating women are at significantly less risk of developing PD. As soon as a woman goes through menopause, her risk of developing PD parallels that of men.

## Should I get blood work to assess my iron status?

A propensity to accumulate iron could be devastating to someone with Parkinsonism. At least once, all men and non-menstruating women should check their ferritin level and iron binding studies. Disorders of iron storage are quite prevalent and easily treated, but they often go undiagnosed. If your binding studies come out within normal limits, and ferritin levels are less than 100, you don't have to worry about iron excess.

## Should I avoid dietary iron?

I recommend consuming red meat sparingly. This recommendation is only in part because of the iron, and mostly because of the well-established health and environmental benefits of limiting beef consumption.

In a prospective study, total iron intake was not associated with an increased risk of Parkinson's disease. Interestingly, low vitamin C and high intake of dietary non-heme iron was associated.[68]../../../../Owner/AppData/Local/Temp/Temp1_Natural Therapies for Parkinson's Disease.zip/Natural Therapies for Parkinson's Disease.html - 57 Non-heme iron refers to plant-sourced iron: rich sources include spinach, kale, and molasses. Given how nutrient-dense these foods are, and the protective antioxidants they also contain, in addition to non-heme iron, I do not advise avoiding them.

# Manganese

Manganese is a metal that has been shown to cause Parkinsonism. This natural element is a well-established neurotoxin.

## What are the most common sources of exposure to manganese?

Symptoms of toxicity usually occur in workers, such as welders and miners, who have been exposed for extended periods of time. The condition of manganese toxicity is called manganism, or welder's disease. Industrial pollution is becoming a more widely recognized source of elevated manganese levels.

Manganese is a naturally occurring element in well water.

- If you are on a well, be sure to use a high-quality water filter and have your water analyzed annually.

## How can I test my manganese levels?

Hair and nail tests accurately assess long-term exposure, providing insight into previous exposures. Urine and blood tests are better methods of assessing and screening for ongoing exposure.

- Doctor's Data provides hair analysis that can inexpensively screen for manganese and many other elements.

## If my manganese levels are elevated, does it mean I don't have Parkinson's disease?

You may well have manganism, resulting in very similar symptoms.

This is a complicated conversation to be had with your neurologist. You should immediately take measures to identify the source of your exposure and work with a physician trained in environmental medicine to reduce your levels.

## *I was diagnosed with Parkinson's disease by a very good neurologist. Can I assume he/she tested me for manganese?*

Unfortunately, no. Screening for manganese levels is not part of a routine diagnostic evaluation of Parkinsonism.

# Marijuana, Cannabis sativa

Marijuana has been used in medicine for thousands of years.

## *Why do people with Parkinson's use marijuana?*

Some individuals perceive an improvement in the symptoms of dyskinesias with marijuana use. An anonymous questionnaire sent to all patients in a Movement Disorder Center revealed that 25% of the 339 respondents had used cannabis. 45.9% of the users described benefit for Parkinson's disease.[69]

In one placebo-controlled study, orally administered marijuana was given to six individuals with Parkinson's disease. Cannabis was well tolerated but resulted in no objective or subjective improvement in Parkinsonism or dyskinesias when administered orally.[70]

## *Does it have to be smoked, or can it be used another way?*

There are dozens of ways to administer cannabinoids, the active ingredients in marijuana. It is most commonly inhaled through water pipes, vaporizers, or the more traditional "joints", or rolled cigarettes. Water pipes and vaporizers are considered to be healthier for your lungs.

Marijuana can also be administered orally, but must first be extracted in a fat. Eating marijuana does alter consciousness, but differently than when it is inhaled. The effects of eating marijuana are usually more long acting.

## Is it safe to use marijuana?

Very little research has been done on the long-term safety of regular use of marijuana. Short-term side effects most commonly include dizziness and increased appetite. Long term concerns surround exposure to inhaled smoke. Marijuana can lead to psychological dependence but carries virtually no risk of physical addiction. Please discuss the risks, and potential benefits, with a physician well versed in the therapeutic value of marijuana.

## Is marijuana legal?

Marijuana use is illegal under federal law, but several states have passed laws permitting the use of medical marijuana. In the United States, its designation as an illicit substance has hindered research efforts and created a stigma for patients.

# Mucuna pruriens, Velvet bean, Cowhage

This legume originated from Indian Ayurvedic medicine. It has traditionally been used as an aphrodisiac and to increase libido. But the seeds of the plant are a naturally occurring source of L-DOPA, identical to synthetic levodopa.

L-DOPA was first isolated from the seeds of the plant in 1937. There is preliminary evidence that some Mucuna preparations might help improve symptom management in PD.

## How does mucuna compare with levodopa/carbidopa for efficacy?

One study compared the efficacy, duration of action, and side effects of these two medicines in eight Parkinson's disease patients. The 30 gram dose of Mucuna led to a considerably faster onset of effect (35 minutes vs. 69 minutes) and longer 'on' time (37 minutes longer). There were no significant differences in dyskinesias or tolerability. The authors concluded:

> The rapid onset of action and longer on time without concomitant increase in dyskinesias on mucuna seed powder formulation suggest that this natural source of L-dopa might possess advantages over conventional L-dopa preparations in the long term management of PD. Assessment of long term efficacy and tolerability in a randomized, controlled study is warranted.[71]

## How does Mucuna work?

Mucuna pruriens cotyledon powder (MPCP) has shown anti-

Parkinson and neuroprotective effects in animal models of Parkinson's disease that are superior to synthetic levodopa.

In a mouse model of PD, Mucuna significantly increased the brain mitochondrial complex-I activity. Unlike synthetic levodopa treatment, it significantly restored the endogenous L-dopa, dopamine, norepinephrine, and serotonin content in the substantia nigra.[72]

While the seeds of the plant do contain L-DOPA, extracts with negligible amounts of L-dopa show significant neuroprotective ability, suggesting that some components other than the L-dopa might be responsible for the anti-Parkinson properties of the seeds.[73] Nicotine adenine dinucleotide (NADH) and coenzyme Q-10, both shown to have therapeutic benefit in Parkinsonism, are present in the seed powder of Mucuna pruriens.

Recently, a study suggested that the ability of MPCP to protect against PD-associated DNA damage may be due to its ability to chelate copper.[74]

## Where can I get MPCP?

Various preparations are available online. It is true that several serious toxicities in recent years have been attributed to Ayurvedic and Chinese medicines. Individuals are encouraged to shop from reputable companies, and when possible, purchase products that are independently certified to be free of contaminants, such as heavy metals.

**Make sure your physician knows you are experimenting with alternative sources of levodopa. You should NOT experiment with Fava beans or Mucuna if:**

- You take a monoamine oxidase inhibitor (MAOI).

Examples include selegiline (Eldepryl, Carbex, deprenyl, Zelapar), rasagiline (Azilect), isocarboxazid (Marplan), phenelzine (Nardil), tranylcypromine (Parnate). MAOIs taken in combination with the above legumes can bring about a dangerous, and sometimes fatal, increase in blood pressure. You must inform your physician if you intend to experiment!

- You have a G6PD deficiency (Favism)

Favism is an inherited genetic disease that causes hemolytic anemia, kidney damage, and possibly death upon consumption of fava beans. G6PD deficiency is rare, occurring mostly among people of Mediterranean, African, and Southeast Asian descent, but others can be affected as well. The disorder is usually detected in childhood, but a blood test can be performed to determine if you are at risk.

# Niacin

In attempts to determine the etiology of Parkinson's disease, Hellenbrand et al. compared the dietary habits of patients vs. a control group; patients were found to have consumed significantly less niacin than controls.[75] In a more recent Swedish study, researchers note that consumption of niacin-containing foods appeared to reduce risk for PD.[76] Finally, in an unpublished study, pellagra was discovered in several patients using levodopa-carbidopa (Iacono et al.).

In 1979, Bender et al. reported the possibility that users of levodopa-carbidopa (Sinemet, Sinemet CR, a medication used to treat the symptoms of PD) could be at risk for both niacin and vitamin B6 deficiencies.[77]

➔ Be sure to take a daily B-complex vitamin. Depending on the quality, your daily dose of B-vitamins may be incorporated into your multivitamin. Check with a health care provider trained in nutritional medicine if you are unsure.

# Tea

For years we have known that consumption of tea seems to protect against the development of PD. Most recently, a study determined that consumption of 3 or more cups per day of tea delayed the age of motor symptoms by 7.7 years![78]

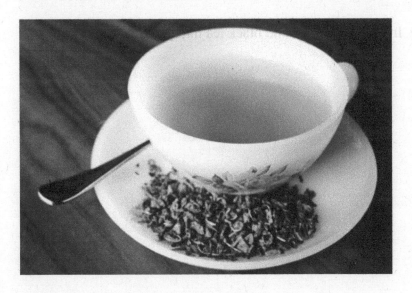

## *Should I drink green tea or black tea?*

Green & black tea come from the same plant, Camellia sinensis. Both are a rich source of antioxidants.

Research results have been mixed as to whether green or black tea is more protective, and the amount required for protection. There is debate as to whether the benefit comes from the caffeine, the antioxidants, or some yet unidentified component(s).

## *Is tea any different than other antioxidants?*

Several studies have demonstrated the ability of green tea to remove iron from the brain. An excessive iron burden in the brain of individuals with PD is not uncommon—iron can promote the generation of toxic free radicals, leading to inflammation and cell death. Tea flavonoids, called catechins, have been shown to possess metal chelating, antioxidant, and anti-inflammatory activities.

➔ Incorporate green and black tea into your diet!

# Vitamin B6

The conversion of L-dopa (levodopa) to dopamine requires B6. Without B6, your body cannot produce its own dopamine, nor can it the medications you're using.

In 1969, 10-15mg of B6 was shown to increase the peripheral conversion of L-dopa to dopamine. By supplementing with B6, levodopa was rapidly converted to dopamine in the gut and bloodstream, reducing the amount of levodopa available to the brain.[79]

B6 is required for the formation of dopamine in both the brain (where we want it) and in the periphery (where we don't).

## *Should I avoid vitamin B6 if I'm taking levodopa?*

No! The brain and body require B6 for function. On the contrary, if you take L-dopa (levodopa, fava beans, etc.), you increase your body's requirement for vitamin B6.

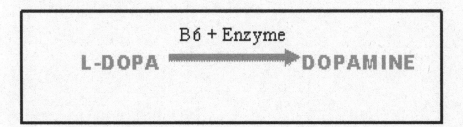

## How much vitamin B6 should I take?

As with all supplement recommendations, it depends on your other medications, the length of time you've been using them, and your current symptoms. Here are the doses I recommend:

5mg/day is sufficient for most people with Parkinson's disease.

10mg/dayx3 months, then reduce to 5mg/day if:

- You have been taking levodopa for more than 5 years.
- Take more than 5 pills/day of levodopa.
- Suffer from depression.

## What are the symptoms of B6 deficiency?

Irritability, depression, confusion, and seizures have all been noted in B6 deficiency. Additional symptoms of deficiency can include inflammation of the tongue, sores or ulcers of the mouth, and ulcers of the skin at the corners of the mouth.

# Vitamin D

Vitamin D is a vitamin and hormone produced from cholesterol inside the body. It remains completely inactive until ultraviolet light (sunlight) penetrates the skin. The roles of vitamin D include protecting against cancer, encouraging the growth of new neurons in the brain, promoting detoxification of toxicants from the brain, and increasing brain antioxidants. Vitamin D is one of the hottest topics in nutrition, and yet it doesn't come from food—it comes from the sun. Individuals who are deficient in vitamin D are more likely to develop PD.[80]

## *What does sunlight have to do with Parkinson's disease?*

Vitamin D has been shown to protect neurons. Studies suggest it plays important roles in the formation and development of neurons and immune system function.[81]

## *Why are so many people deficient in vitamin D?*

Vitamin D normally comes from sunlight. Grey skies, days spent covered with clothing or indoors, distance from the equator, and cloud cover all contribute to inadequate vitamin D levels. As the US population spends more time indoors—at the office, playing video games, watching TV—less time is spent absorbing this essential nutrient!

## *Should I have my vitamin D levels checked?*

Yes! Everyone should be screened for vitamin D deficiency as least

121

once yearly, and preferably in the winter. If you have been diagnosed with a neurological disease or have a family history of neurological diseases, you should have your level checked several times per year to ensure adequate levels.

→ 25-OH vitamin D is the name of the blood test for assessing vitamin D status.

## What should my level of vitamin D (25-OH vitamin D) be?

While it is clear that vitamin D deficiency is unhealthy, researchers have not yet figured out what blood level is optimal.

→ Keep vitamin D levels between 50-8 ng/mL.

## Is vitamin D dangerous?

Vitamin D is one of the few fat-soluble vitamins and is associated with a risk of toxicity, even death! Under the care of a physician, one should not be afraid to supplement with vitamin D. In fact, most US doctors are quite conservative in their dosing, often taking several months to correct a deficiency.

→ Do not take vitamin D doses above 2000 IU/day without a blood test and supervision of your health care provider.

## I read that vitamin D3 was preferable to vitamin D2, but my doctor gave me a prescription for vitamin D2. Why?

Vitamin D3 is sourced from lanolin and is the most biologically available form of vitamin D. Unfortunately, the only prescription form available (covered by your insurance) is vitamin D2. It is usually given as a megadose of 50,000 IU once or twice weekly.

An alternative dosing regime is to take 6000-10,000 IU/day of vitamin D3. This provides the more highly-absorbed form of the vitamin in doses that mimic exposure to the sun. (Sunbathing will generate about 10,000 IU/day.)

→ Do not combine your doctor's prescription for D2 with over-the-counter D3! This is how one develops toxicity! If you'd prefer the D3 form, discuss this with your health care provider.

## Is there ever a time when vitamin D2 is preferable to D3?

D2 is sourced from plants, and as such, is often preferred by vegans. Also, since vitamin D2 only requires dosing 1-2 times/week, it is sometimes preferable with patients who have a hard time remembering to take the daily dose.

## Isn't vitamin D important for bone health?

Osteoporosis and osteopenia are common in Parkinson's disease, affecting up to 91% of women and 61% of men. Because of balance issues and episodes of freezing associated with medications, patients are at increased risk for falls and fractures.[82]

→ To evaluate the health of your bones: Ask your doctor for a DEXA scan every other year.

# VI. ENCOURAGING OPTIMAL HEALTH

## a. Promoting Health as a Treatment Strategy

The way the game of PD is currently played is largely defensive. The most commonly prescribed drugs help control symptoms in a diseased brain. None of the conventional therapies has as its target:

- to slow or stop destruction of the diseased area;
- to improve health of underlying tissues;
- to provide ingredients for healthy function.

Although genetics and environmental factors contribute to the development of PD, emerging evidence suggests that the majority of individuals with PD have mitochondrial dysfunction and increased free radicals.

The mitochondria are the part of the cell responsible for energy production, the "powerhouse of the cell" (recall 10th grade biology). If the cell is unable to produce enough energy to sustain it, the cell subsequently dies, producing free radicals and inflammation in the surrounding tissue. This is exactly what happens in the substantia nigra of patients with PD.

Free radicals are unpaired electrons that create havoc in surrounding tissues. Sources of excessive free radicals include metals in the blood (iron, mercury, manganese, copper, aluminum),

125

smoked & charred foods, alcohol, fried foods, hydrogenated oils, and air pollution.

Here are some things we can definitely do:

1. **Neuroprotection:**

   Researchers are attempting to identify the best way to protect the neurons from dying and optimize the health of the remaining ones. In the meantime, it seems easy enough to limit the things known to create free radicals and increase things known to contribute to the health of the mitochondria and surrounding tissue.

2. **Increase survival of neurons:**

   Through calorie restriction and exercise.

3. **Increase production of dopamine**

4. **Ensure adequate co-factors for synthesis (tyrosine, B-6, etc.)**

5. **Decrease the accumulation of alpha-synuclein**

   Vitamin A, beta-carotene, and coenzyme Q10.[83]

6. **Minimize comorbid conditions**

   Constipation (See Section entitled: Constipation)

   Osteoporosis (See Section entitled: Vitamin D)

Cardiovascular disease (See Sections entitled: Homocysteine, Calorie restriction, Exercise, Fish Oil)

Depression (See Section entitled: DHA)

## 7. Symptom Management

Allopathic medicine works well.

Bradykinesia (slowness), rigidity, tremor, and handwriting have been shown to be improved with choline, Mucuna, and fava beans.

Nutritional L-dopa (See Section entitled: Fava beans)

## 8. Decrease medication side effects

Dyskinesias (See Section entitled: DHA/Fish oil)

On-Off/Wearing off: (See Section entitled: Citicoline)

Anti-nutrient properties (See Section entitled: Homocysteine)

## 9. Increase survival of neurons

Lipoic acid and acetyl-L-carntine

Turmeric and green tea

127

# b. Working with a trained provider

There are dozens of options for individuals with Parkinsonism. Becoming aware of them can leave one's head spinning. It seems like the more we learn, the less we know. Managing side effects, drug-nutrient interactions, and dosing schedules is virtually a full-time job.

The websites below offer referral recommendations for physicians trained in complementary, alternative, and integrative medicine (CAIM).

**Naturopathic doctors**: www.naturopathic.org

Naturopathic doctors (ND) hold clinical doctorates and are licensed primary care providers in many US states. If you are fortunate enough to live in a licensed state, take advantage of it! Naturopathic medical schools are the only medical schools in the country that, from day one of the education, stress the holistic principles and differences between individuals.

**Orthomolecular physicians**: www.orthomolecular.org

Orthomolecular medicine is studied and practiced by a diverse group of practitioners with the common interest of studying and optimizing the function of the body. MDs, NDs, PhDs, dentists, among others, from all over the world, identify with the cause, Therapeutic nutrition based upon biochemical individuality.

**American College for the Advancement in Medicine**: www.acam.org

ACAM is an association dedicated to educating conventional

physicians on the latest findings and emerging procedures in complementary, alternative, and integrative medicine (CAIM).

# c. On the Use of Supplements

It is absolutely essential to use only supplements from reputable sources. It is very difficult to know a reputable source, as there are very few federally regulated guidelines. In addition to concerns about safety, product contamination, and interactions with other medications, most people want to know that they are not wasting their money.

The highest-quality lines of supplements are sold only to licensed health care providers and pharmacists. Some of the highest quality supplements include Douglas Laboratories, Pharmax, Thorne, and Vital Nutrients. These companies provide independent quality analysis and assurance that their products are free of contaminants. Over the counter supplements, unfortunately, do not always contain what the label says they do.

> Patients often comment that switching brands of a particular supplement changes their response. This is a common experience with coenzyme Q-10 and fish oil.

Be clear why you are taking the supplements you are taking—to protect the neurons, to decrease symptoms, or to prevent medication side effects. It is more difficult to determine efficacy of "neuroprotection." We can't know how you would have progressed had you done something different. If your disease is not progressing, you are doing it right!

# d. Combining Conventional & Alternative Therapies

Most practitioners have the same common goal—to improve brain function. The only difference is in the approach we each take.

## What will my neurologist think?

That depends on your neurologist. Personally, I have never met an irrational neurologist. Most seem pretty straight-forward and intrigued by thought-provoking concepts. Most sincerely want to improve the health of their patients. Many doctors have had the experience of watching patients spend way too much time and money on hoaxes and scams. Give a copy of this book to your neurologist—it has been designed to convey the scientific rationale behind the most commonly used natural therapies in Parkinsonism. It is intended to open dialogue.

## What should I tell my provider?

When you start a new medicine, natural or pharmaceutical, you should tell your providers about it. Once a year, you should provide your doctor with the following information:

| Start date | Medication | Dose | Frequency | Brand | Reason | Prescribing Provider | Stop date |
|---|---|---|---|---|---|---|---|
|  |  |  |  |  |  |  |  |
|  |  |  |  |  |  |  |  |
|  |  |  |  |  |  |  |  |
|  |  |  |  |  |  |  |  |
|  |  |  |  |  |  |  |  |

# My physician does not have much experience with CAM therapies—what should I say to him/her?

For your safety, it is important to tell your physician what you are taking. There are many interactions between pharmaceutical medications and the CAM therapies outlined in this book. It is your physician's responsibility to be informed about the medications you are taking and how they may interact with those being prescribed.

**Worst-case scenario:** Occasionally I come across a patient who insists their doctor is not open to any form of alternative medicine and is dismissive when the topic is broached.

# My doctor does not believe in alternative medicine.

This is absurd. We are talking about science, not faith—it's not about "belief." If this really does come out of your provider's mouth, an appropriate response might be, "You don't believe what about alternative medicine?" or "How are you defining alternative medicine?" The goal is to open dialogue and evolve a mutual understanding.

# My doctor told me that alternative medicine doesn't work.

The field Complementary and Alternative Medicine (CAM) is huge. It includes everything from nutrition to acupuncture, music and art therapy, herbal medicines, and exposure to magnetic fields. Such an oversimplified comment, implying that alternative medicine is one thing, reflects tremendous ignorance. Which therapy for which disease? Under which conditions?

## *What if he/she insists I not use CAM therapies?*

First, try to understand where he/she is coming from—is he discouraging fish oil because you have a bleeding disorder? Is she discouraging coenzyme Q10 because she thinks it's not a good use of your money? Is she telling you not to eat fava beans because you are on a high-dose MAO-B inhibitor and have G6PD deficiency? Your doctor may have a very good reason for his/her opinions: make sure you understand why a therapy is being discouraged.

If your doctor does not have a good reason, but discourages all therapies that are unconventional, you should find a new doctor. If your doctor does not know how to cure your disease, he/she should be actively looking for new ideas, treatments, strategies, and therapies. A doctor who does not know how to cure you, and refuses to entertain new ideas to that end, should be rapidly replaced.

Your doctor should not be expected to become an authority in CAM or even take interest in it. Everybody has interests, and complementary medicine is not for everyone. Your doctor should be able to refer you to a trusted authority on the subject in your community and be willing to collaborate with other providers when necessary.

# e. Drug-Nutrient Interactions

### 1. Levodopa, carbidopa/levodopa, C/L, Sinemet

- Depletes folic acid

- C/L decreases the ability of folic acid to be absorbed across
  the gut, into the bloodstream

- C/L increases the body's utilization of, and thus requirement
  for, folic acid

  → If you take levodopa, take 400-800mcg/day of folic acid

- Competes with protein for absorption

Levodopa competes with the five large neutral amino acids for
carriers, both in the gut and at the blood-brain barrier.[84] Thus, high
protein meals have the potential to cause an erratic response to
levodopa.

  → DO NOT AVOID PROTEIN! The goal is to have your
    medicine work for you, not you working for your
    medicine.

  → Take levodopa 30 minutes before meals, especially meals
    high in protein (meat, beans, and nuts).

- Nausea is a common side effect of levodopa.

Balancing nutrition and medications is difficult enough, nausea
makes it worse! While carbohydrates usually do help nausea, most
of them are void of nutrients and not a habit you want to get into
with each dose of levodopa. For most people, the nausea is worst in

the morning, or when taken on an empty stomach. The goal is to find carbohydrates and fats that are a good source of nutrition to eat with your medication.

→ Try eating a 1/2 banana, oatmeal, or some dolmas with your medications if you find yourself experiencing nausea.

If you don't experience nausea, it's fine to take levodopa on an empty stomach.

- Increases requirement for vitamin B6

Vitamin B6 is necessary to convert levodopa to dopamine. In 1969, 10-15mg B6 was shown to increase conversion of L-dopa to dopamine in the bloodstream, before it could get to the brain.[85] If you avoid vitamin B6, you will also inhibit your brain's ability to convert L-dopa to dopamine! Your efforts to increase levodopa efficacy will backfire!

→ Make sure the body has all the vitamin B6 it needs, and then adjust your dose of medication appropriately.

- Raises homocysteine

Homocysteine is an amino acid produced by the body; levels go up when one becomes deficient in vitamins B6, B12, folic acid, or betaine. Levodopa has been shown to raise homocysteine levels, which have been associated with a more rapidly progressing disease and a greater likelihood of cognitive symptoms. (See Section entitled: Homocysteine)

→ Take a B-complex vitamin daily if you take levodopa.

➔ Get your blood homocysteine levels checked annually. Make sure they stay below 10 mmol/L, which is easily accomplished with B-vitamin supplementation.

➔ Iron supplements can reduce availability of levodopa.

When patients were simultaneously administered 325mg ferrous sulfate and levodopa, there was a 47% decrease in peak plasma concentrations of levodopa. Some patients experienced a loss of clinical efficacy.[86]

➔ Iron supplements should only be taken by individuals with Parkinsonism if they have an iron deficiency identified by their health care provider.

➔ When necessary, iron supplements should be taken with a protein-containing meal, away from levodopa.

This doesn't mean the C/L is "bad." It means that for as long as you are taking C/L you need to take additional measures to ensure adequate nutritional status and safeguard against side effects. The information above should allow you to use levodopa to control your symptoms safely.

## 2. MAO-B Inhibitors

Monoamine oxidase B acts in the brain to break down dopamine. Therefore, preventing it from functioning is a therapeutic strategy for PD treatment. You should know if you are on one of these drugs, as they come with certain necessary precautions! If you are unsure, ask your doctor. Examples of MAO-B inhibitors used in the treatment of PD are selegeline and rasagaline (Azilect).

➔ Be aware of tyramine in foods.

Inhibition of MAO enzymes can lead to life-threatening hypertensive crisis when tyramine-containing foods or drugs are consumed. The new generation of MAO-inhibitors used in PD poses less risk than the first generation, but caution is still recommended.

Tyramine-containing foods to limit if you are on a MAO-B inhibitor:
- Air-dried or fermented meats
- Pickled herring
- Fava beans
- Soy beans and soy products
- Aged cheeses
- Red wine
- Non-pasteurized beer

There are MAO interactions with other pharmaceuticals, such as the ingredients are commonly found in cold/sinus medications. Drugs to avoid include pseudoephedrine, phenylephrine, phenylproanalamine, and ephedrine. Please ask your pharmacist for a more complete list.

### 3. Statins

The class of drugs known as statins are commonly used in the US to reduce cholesterol levels. They work by reducing the function of the liver enzyme, HMGCoA reductase. This enzyme also happens to be the body's source of coenzyme-Q10. (See Sections entitled: Coenzyme-Q10, Cholesterol)

➔ If you have elevated cholesterol, save statins as a very last resort in cholesterol management.

➔ If you must use a statin, be sure to supplement with additional coenzyme Q-10 and ensure that your total cholesterol levels do not fall below 160.

## Ways to reduce cholesterol without statins

- Exercise
- Fiber
- Fish oil

- Dairy
- Red meat
- Saturated fat

# VII. PREVENTION: Recommendations for Children of Parkinson's Patients

This chapter is dedicated to the relatives of those with PD, a vulnerable and neglected group.

The cure for Parkinsonism is prevention. Studies suggest that more than 50% of the mass of the substantia nigra has been lost by the time the first symptoms of Parkinsonism appear. Loss of smell and constipation may be early symptoms.

The more brain that has been lost, it stands to reason that it will be more difficult to impart notable change. The early one gets started on the task of preventing and slowing the disease, the better.

Patients are often disheartened to learn that, at diagnosis, they have already lost about 50% of the affected part of their brain. I encourage you to consider how amazing the human brain is—that it can lose 50% of one area, without consequence to the individual. So what if some brain mass has been lost? Let's figure out how to improve the function of remaining neurons and see if they can't pick of the slack for what's been lost.

## Am I at increased risk of developing PD if one of my parents has PD?

Yes. A family history of PD is the single strongest predictor of developing this disease.

## Why do some people with a family history develop PD, and others do not?

139

Our fate is only partially determined by our genetic profile. What genes get expressed, and how well the body functions, depends on the environment we expose ourselves to.

You can't change the hand of cards you're dealt. The game is how best to play them.

## Are there things I can do to decrease my risk of developing PD?

While no study has investigated this question yet, it stands to reason that changing your environment has the potential to influence your risk of disease.

## What are my options for prevention?

The conventional therapies for PD—pharmacotherapy and surgery—are not indicated for asymptomatic individuals. The only thing these drugs are believed to do is treat the symptoms. Thus, they become useless if one doesn't have symptoms.

Many of the therapies covered in this book are easy to incorporate into one's diet, lifestyle, etc. and come with very little risk or expense.

→ Several studies have shown that individuals who consume more dairy are more likely to develop PD. I recommend that all children of PD patients avoid dairy.

→ Several studies show that drinking tea is protective against the development of PD. I recommend that all children of PD patients drink more green tea.

## *Why don't we study prevention?*

The late onset of Parkinsonian symptoms makes it very difficult to study. Researchers estimate the disease process has been underway for 5-10 years by the time the first symptoms appear.

And even if we could predict who will develop PD, there is no conventional therapy to offer them. Given the side effects and limitations of dopamine repletion therapy, the currently available PD medications are useless for any significant amount of prevention.

# a. DIET

- Avoid dairy.
- Eat plenty of fruits, vegetables, fish, legumes, whole grain, and poultry.
- Drink green and black tea.
- Drink coffee and alcohol only in moderation.

**Accessory nutrients:**

- Turmeric is a source of curcumin.
- Egg yolks are a rich source of choline.

# b. SUPPLEMENTS

- Multivitamin: high-quality capsules.
- Fish oil: 1000mg/day of EPA + DHA.
- Coenzyme Q10: 100mg/day.

# c. LIFESTYLE

- Avoid pesticides: Eat organic. Wash non-organic food thoroughly before consuming.
- Do not have your clothes dry-cleaned. If you must, let them off-gas outside for several days before wearing them.
- Use a high-quality water filter if you are on a well.

# d. ANNUAL TESTING

- Vitamin D (25-OH vitamin D): Optimal range: 50-100.
- Homocysteine: Optimal range: 5-10.
- SpectraCell Intracellular Nutritional Analysis.
- Ensure adequacy of coenyzme Q10, glutathione, vitamin E, and other antioxidants.

> Early detection creates greater opportunity for prevention.
> Awareness always increases your options.

Markers that put someone at high risk for developing PD:
- Family history of PD
- Loss of sense of smell
- Constipation
- REM sleep disorder
- Dementia
- Abnormalities in SPECT imaging of the heart

With the advance of genetic medicine, it is only a matter of time before carriers of particular genes will also qualify as 'at risk' individuals.

144

# VIII. Recipes

Eating is an art. Like any other game of strategy, the challenge is to identify and provide what is required and avoid what is detrimental.

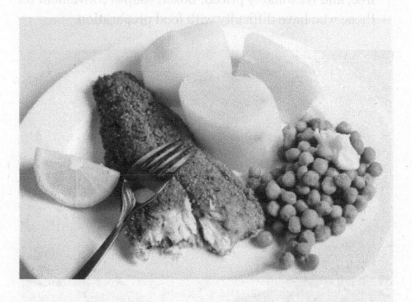

But food is not just about nutrition. Food is cultural, ceremonial, psychological, sensual, and practical. What, and how, we eat shapes our community and is shaped by our community.

The learning curve is steep. Learn to cook with high-ORAC spices: (See Chapter: Antioxidants)

## BREAKFAST IDEAS

Oatmeal

Instant is fine. Add cinnamon liberally—it doubles as medicine!

Soup

Soup is an easy way to get vegetables and beans into the diet, and easy to digest. Boxed soup is available organic, dairy free, and reasonably priced. Boxed soup is convenient for those who have difficulty with food preparation.

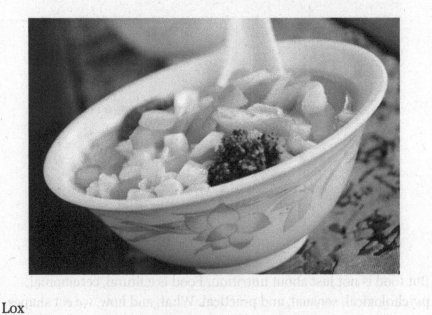

Lox

Smoked salmon is delicious and nutritious. Lox counts as a serving of omega-3 fatty acids, which are necessary for brain function.

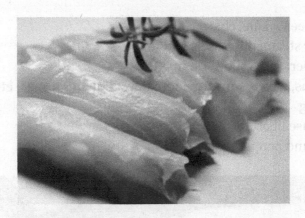

Pea, Rice, Hemp, or Soy Protein powder

> Protein powder is ideal for people who prefer to skip breakfast. Taken 30-45 minutes following medications, it's an easily absorbed and nutrient-dense meal substitute. Soy makes some people bloat, so be aware. Whey protein, the most common in stores, is derived from dairy and thus contraindicated in PD.

Eggs

> Eggs cooked under water are healthier than those exposed to air during preparation—hard-boiled and poached are recommended. The yolk has specific nutritional value in PD, as it is a rich source of choline. Frittatas are a great delivery mechanism for vegetables!

FRITTATA (Scrambled Egg Pizza)

Ingredients:

2 tbsp vegetable oil (from a glass bottle): canola, olive, safflower
1 onion

1 bunch greens: kale, chard, spinach
10 leftover steamed Brussels sprouts
1 bell pepper: red, yellow, or green
mushrooms, olives, sun-dried tomatoes, Italian sausage, etc. to
one's liking
Sea salt—use liberally
Fresh ground pepper- use liberally

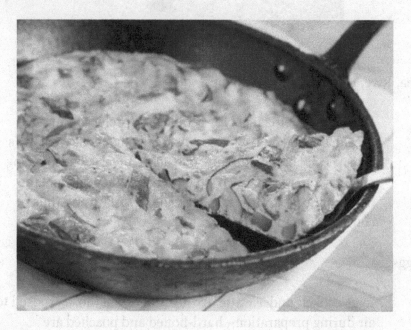

Instructions:

Preheat the broiler in the oven. Use a cast iron skillet suitable for
both stove and oven.

Sauté onions and greens on the stove, when it reduces in size, add
remaining veggies.

When they start to soften, pour in 6-8 scrambled eggs. Add high
quality salt and pepper, as both of these have nutritional value when

used fresh. The more herbs and spices you add, the healthier it becomes.

Mix scrambled eggs and veggies together quickly and cover—no more stirring. Let the egg cook from the bottom, not unlike an omelet. As soon as the edges begin to harden, move it to the top shelf of the oven (set on broil) for 2-3 minutes.

Remove as soon as the top starts to brown, and let it cook for 10 minutes. Fresh salsa on top can't be beat, but ketchup will do.

Makes great leftovers.

Slow cooker

> Slow cookers are terribly convenient for those who want good food, cooked from home, and don't want to spend the day preparing it.

Pot roast

> Easy to prepare and easily digestible. Meat should be grass-fed, free-range, and hormone free. Throw in large chunks of onions, carrots, and potatoes. Add water, cover, and cook for 6+ hours.

Snacks

> Fruit + nuts

> Apple and peanut butter

> Rice cake + cashew butter

# LUNCH IDEAS

Split pea soup

> Another great way to increase consumption of legumes. Canned and boxed soups are tasty and readily available, but it's pretty easy to make in the slow cooker, too. Soak peas overnight and rinse. Add to slow cooker with chopped carrots, onions, and spices.

Taco salad

> Sauté an onion, ground turkey and taco seasoning- let cool once cooked. Chop lettuce, peppers, tomatoes, avocado, olives, etc. and mix together with meat and French dressing. Add crumbled corn chips just prior to eating, so they don't get soggy.

Dolmas

> A Mediterranean dish—rice, olive oil, garlic, and lemon juice rolled up in a grape leaf. A great source of healthy oils. The 'good fats' make it satiating. Because they are low in protein, they tend not to interfere with medications.

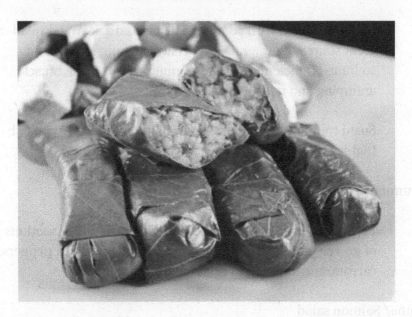

Sushi + seaweed salad

Japanese restaurants are a rich source of nutrient rich foods. Most foods on the menu are dairy-free, and they serve a lot of omega-3 rich fish.

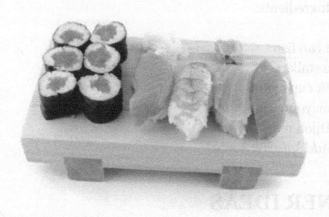

Start your meal with edamame beans and a seaweed salad- a great source of minerals, especially calcium, iodine, and sodium. (Deficiencies of these minerals can cause muscle cramping and neurological symptoms.)

Sushi rolls are available vegetarian and also come with fish that is either cooked or raw, to your preference.

## Hummus + veggies

Premade hummus is available in most refrigerated sections of grocery stores. Cut up cucumbers, tomatoes, bell peppers, carrots, and any other vegetable for dipping.

## Tuna/ Salmon salad

Canned fish is convenient, inexpensive, and a source of omega-3 fatty acids that are good for the brain. Canned salmon often comes with the bones inside; softened by the juices, these bones are an excellent source of calcium.

Ingredients:

1 can fish
2 stalks celery
¼ cup onions
mayonnaise
Dijon mustard
*Add spices & herbs!*

# DINNER IDEAS

Chili

Beans and spices are medicinal in PD!

Veggie burgers

There is nothing wrong with meat and the occasional burger made from flesh. Veggie burgers need not replace meat burgers. They are in the freezer section of most stores, inexpensive, convenient, and commonly made from beans- another easy way to meet nutritional goals in PD.

Grilled:

Marinated portabella mushroom
Asparagus- grilled
Polenta- on the stove
Crab cakes/ Salmon cakes
Chicken + Coconut milk + Coconut + Turmeric

# XI. GUIDELINES FOR EATING WITH PARKINSONISM

- Choose nutrient-dense foods.

  → If the food you're about to eat is not a rich source of nutrients, don't eat it!

- No dairy.
- High fiber.
- Lots of water.
- High antioxidants:
  o Brightly-colored fruits and vegetables
  o Green & black tea
  o Beans/legumes
- Fish—5 servings per week.
- Fava beans.
- Moderate protein consumption:
  o Mostly from beans and poultry.
- Spices—turmeric, cinnamon, cloves.
- Egg yolks (choline source)—6/week.

## *Why seasonal?*

There is an ancient understanding of the relationship between food, environment, and us called Macrobiotics. Its teachings are simple: eat with respect for what's around you, be moderate, cook and eat with intention. Strawberries only taste good in early summer, pumpkin pie only in the fall.

# *Why organic?*

There is no question that exposure to pesticides is a risk factor for developing Parkinsonism. Avoiding pesticides seems like a good idea for a person with Parkinsonism, or anyone seeking brain health. One very good way to avoid exposure is to not spray our food with them.

# NATURAL THERAPIES FOR PD

## To protect neurons and encourage function

- Alpha-lipoic acid
- Calorie restriction
- Coenzyme Q10
- Creatine
- Glutathione
- Fish oil
- Tea, green or black
- Turmeric
- Vitamin D

## For symptoms
- Fava beans
- Mucuna

## To limit/reduce the amount of levodopa you require
- Citicoline

## To reduce medication side effects
- Fish oil
- Folic acid, vitamin B6, vitamin B12, betaine (homocystrol-lowering nutrients)

## Avoid environmental and dietary neurotoxins
- Aluminum
- Aspartame
- Copper
- Dairy
- Dry cleaning chemicals
- Manganese
- Pesticides: Eat organic and don't spray your yard

# X. References

[1] Stacy, M. and J. Jankovic. Differential diagnosis of Parkinson's disease and the parkinsonism plus syndromes. Neurol Clin 1992;10(2): 341-59.

[2] Olanow, C.W., M.B. Stern, and K. Sethi. The scientific and clinical basis for the treatment of Parkinson disease. Neurology 2009;72(21 Suppl 4): S1-136.

[3] Jellinger, K.A. Lewy body-related alpha-synucleinopathy in the aged human brain. J Neural Transm 2004;111(10-11): 1219-35.

[4] Olanow, C.W., et al. Lewy-body formation is an aggresome-related process: a hypothesis. Lancet Neurol, 2004;3(8): 496-503.

[5] Braak, H., et al. Stages in the development of Parkinson's disease-related pathology. Cell Tissue Res 2004;318(1): 121-34.

[6] Ono, K. and M. Yamada. Vitamin A potently destabilizes preformed alpha-synuclein fibrils in vitro: implications for Lewy body diseases. Neurobiol Dis 2007;25(2): 446-54.

[7] Ono, K. and M. Yamada. Antioxidant compounds have potent anti-fibrillogenic and fibril-destabilizing effects for alpha-synuclein fibrils in vitro. J Neurochem 2006;97(1): 105-15.

[8] Wang YH, Yan F, Zhang WB, et al. An investigation of vitamin B12 deficiency in elderly inpatients in neurology department. Neurosci Bull Aug 2009;25(4):209-215.

[9] Gao X CH, Fung TT, et al. A Prospective study of dietary pattern and risk of Parkinson disease. Am J Clin Nutr 2007;86: 1486-1494.

[10] Schelosky L, Raffauf C, Jendroska K, Poewe W. Kava and dopamine antagonism. J Neurol Neurosurg Psychiatry May 1995;58(5):639-640.

[11] Shen W, Liu K, Tian C, et al. R-alpha-lipoic acid and acetyl-L-carnitine complementarily promote mitochondrial biogenesis in murine 3T3-L1 adipocytes. Diabetologia 2008;51(1): 165-174.

[12] Bilska A, Dubiel M, Sokolowska-Jezewicz M, Lorenc-Koci E, and Wlodek L. Alpha-lipoic acid differently affects the reserpine-

induced oxidative stress in the striatum and prefrontal cortex of rat brain. Neuroscience Jun 8 2007;146(4): 1758-1771.

[13] Shen W, Liu K, Tian C, et al. R-alpha-lipoic acid and acetyl-L-carnitine complementarily promote mitochondrial biogenesis in murine 3T3-L1 adipocytes. Diabetologia Jan 2008;51(1): 165-174.

[14] Liu J. 2008. Neurochem Res 2008; 33(1):194.

[15] Milanese M, Lkhayat MI, and Zatta P. Inhibitory effect of aluminum on dopamine beta-hydroxylase from bovine adrenal gland. J Trace Elem Med Biol 2001;15(2-3): 139-141.

[16] Uversky VN, Li J, Bower K, Fink AL. Synergistic effects of pesticides and metals on the fibrillation of alpha-synuclein: implications for Parkinson's disease. Neurotoxicology Oct 2002;23(4-5): 527-536.

[17] Graves AB, White E, Koepsell TD, Reifler BV, van Belle G, and Larson EB. The association between aluminum-containing products and Alzheimer's disease. J Clin Epidemiol 1990;43(1): 35-44.

[18] Campbell A, Bondy SC. Aluminum as a toxicant. Toxicol Ind Health Aug 2002;18(7): 309-320.

[19] Baker SK, Tarnopolsky MA. Targeting cellular energy production in neurological disorders. Expert Opin Investig Drugs Oct 2003;12(10): 1655-1679.

[20] Beal MF. Bioenergetic approaches for neuroprotection in Parkinson's disease. Ann Neurol 2003;53(Suppl 3): S39-47.

[21] Kidd PM. Neurodegeneration from mitochondrial insufficiency: nutrients, stem cells, growth factors, and prospects for brain rebuilding using integrative management. Altern Med Rev Dec 2005;10(4): 268-293.

[22] Calabrese V, Cornelius C, Mancuso C, et al. Cellular stress response: a novel target for chemoprevention and nutritional neuroprotection in aging, neurodegenerative disorders and longevity. Neurochem Res Dec 2008;33(12): 2444-2471.

[23] Ono K, Yamada M. Vitamin A potently destabilizes preformed alpha-synuclein fibrils in vitro: implications for Lewy body diseases. Neurobiol Dis Feb 2007;25(2): 446-454.

[24] Ibid.

[25] Unlu NZ, Bohn T, Clinton SK, Schwartz SJ. Carotenoid absorption from salad and salsa by humans is enhanced by the addition of avocado or avocado oil. J Nutr Mar 2005;135(3): 431-436.

[26] Love R. Calorie restriction may be neuroprotective in AD and PD. Lancet Neurol. Feb 2005;4(2):84.

[27] Maswood N, Young J, Tilmont E, et al. Caloric restriction increases neurotrophic factor levels and attenuates neurochemical and behavioral deficits in a primate model of Parkinson's disease. Proc Natl Acad Sci USA Dec 28 2004;101(52): 18171-18176.

[28] Mattson MP. Will caloric restriction and folate protect against AD and PD? Neurology Feb25 2003;60(4): 690-695.

[29] Bruce-Keller AJ, Umberger G, McFall R, and Mattson MP. Food restriction reduces brain damage and improves behavioral outcome following excitotoxic and metabolic insults. Ann Neurol Jan 1999;45(1): 8-15.

[30] Higdon J DV, Hagen TM. L-Carnitine. 2009; http://lpi.oregonstate.edu/infocenter/othernuts/carnitine/.

[31] Zhang, H, Jia H, and Liu, J. et al. Combined R-alpha-lipoic acid and acetyl-L-carnatine exerts efficient preventative effects in a cellular model of Parkinson's Disease. J Cell Mol Med 2008: 1-20.

[32] Kaikkonen J NK, et al. Determinants of plasma coenzyme Q10 in humans. FEBS Lett. 1999.

[33] Reiss AB SK, et al. Cholesterol in neurologic disorders of the elderly. 2004.

[34] Teunissen CE, Lutjohann D, von Bergmann K, et al. Combination of serum markers related to several mechanisms in Alzheimer's disease. Neurobiol Aging Nov 2003;24(7): 893-902.

[35] Sohmiya M, Tanaka M, Aihara Y, Okamoto K. Structural changes in the midbrain with aging and Parkinson's disease: an MRI study. Neurobiol Aging Apr 2004;25(4): 449-453.

[36] de Lau LM, Koudstaal PJ, Hofman A, Breteler MM. Serum cholesterol levels and the risk of Parkinson's disease. Am J Epidemiol Nov 15 2006;164(10): 998-1002.

[37] de Lau LM, Stricker BH, Breteler MM. Serum cholesterol, use of lipid-lowering drugs, and risk of Parkinson disease. Mov Disord Oct 15 2007;22(13): 1985.

[38] Manyam BV, Giacobini E, Colliver JA. Cerebrospinal fluid choline levels are decreased in Parkinson's disease. Ann Neurol Jun 1990;27(6): 683-685.

[39] Cubells JM, Hernando C. Clinical trial on the use of cytidine diphosphate choline in Parkinson's disease. Clin Ther 1988;10(6): 664-671.

[40] Agnoli A, Ruggieri S, Denaro A, Bruno G. New strategies in the management of Parkinson's disease: a biological approach using a phospholipid precursor (CDP-choline). Neuropsychobiology 1982;8(6): 289-296.

[41] Eberhardt R, Birbamer G, Gerstenbrand F, Rainer E, Traegner H. Citicoline in the treatment of Parkinson's disease Clin Ther Nov-Dec 1990;12(6): 489-495.

[42] Shults CW, Oakes D, Kieburtz K, et al. Effects of coenzyme Q10 in early Parkinson disease: evidence of slowing of the functional decline. Arch Neurol Oct 2002;59(10): 1541-1550.

[43] Shults CW, Flint Beal M, Song D, and Fontaine D. Pilot trial of high dosages of coenzyme Q10 in patients with Parkinson's disease. Exp Neurol Aug 2004;188(2): 491-494.

[44] Abbott RD, Petrovitch H, White LR, et al. Frequency of bowel movements and the future risk of Parkinson's disease. Neurology Aug 14 2001;57(3): 456-462.

[45] Petrovitch H, Abbott RD, Ross GW, et al. Bowel movement frequency in late-life and substantia nigra neuron density at death. Mov Disord Feb 15 2009;24(3): 371-376.

[46] Bender A, Koch W, Elstner M, et al. Creatine supplementation in Parkinson disease: a placebo-controlled randomized pilot trial. Neurology Oct 10 2006;67(7): 1262-1264.

[47] A randomized, double-blind, futility clinical trial of creatine and minocycline in early Parkinson disease. Neurology Mar 14 2006;66(5): 664-671.

[48] Sun AY, Wang Q, Simonyi A, Sun GY. Botanical phenolics and brain health. Neuromolecular Med 2008;10(4): 259-274.

[49] Agnoli A, Ruggieri S, Denaro A, Bruno G. New strategies in the management of Parkinson's disease: a biological approach using a phospholipid precursor (CDP-choline). Neuropsychobiology 1982;8(6): 289-296.

[50] Jagatha B, Mythri RB, Vali S, Bharath MM. Curcumin treatment alleviates the effects of glutathione depletion in vitro and in vivo: therapeutic implications for Parkinson's disease explained via in silico studies. Free Radic Biol Med Mar 1 2008;44(5): 907-917.

[51] Sethi P, Jyoti A, Hussain E, and Sharma D. Curcumin attenuates aluminium-induced functional neurotoxicity in rats. Pharmacol Biochem Behav Jul 2009;93(1): 31-39.

[52] Park M, Ross GW, Petrovitch H, et al. Consumption of milk and calcium in midlife and the future risk of Parkinson disease. Neurology Mar 22 2005;64(6): 1047-1051.

[53] Chen H, O'Reilly E, McCullough ML, et al. Consumption of dairy products and risk of Parkinson's disease. Am J Epidemiol May 1 2007;165(9): 998-1006.

[54] Chen H, Zhang SM, Hernan MA, Willett WC, Ascherio A. Diet and Parkinson's disease: a potential role of dairy products in men. Ann Neurol Dec 2002;52(6): 793-801.

[55] Samadi P, Gregoire L, Rouillard C, Bedard PJ, Di Paolo T, and Levesque D. Docosahexaenoic acid reduces levodopa-induced dyskinesias in 1-methyl-4-phenyl-1,2,3,6-tetrahydropyridine monkeys. Ann Neurol Feb 2006;59(2): 282-288.

[56] Ibid.

[57] Martin HL, Teismann P. Glutathione—a review on its role and significance in Parkinson's disease. FASEB J Jun 19 2009.

[58] Sechi G, Deledda MG, Bua G, et al. Reduced intravenous glutathione in the treatment of early Parkinson's disease. Prog Neuropsychopharmacol Biol Psychiatry Oct 1996;20(7): 1159-1170.

[59] Strang RR. The Association of Gastro-Duodenal Ulceration and Parkinson's Disease. Med J Aust Jun 5 1965;1(23): 842-843.

[60] Szabo S. Dopamine disorder in duodenal ulceration. Lancet Oct 27 1979;2(8148): 880-882.

[61] Dobbs RJ, Dobbs SM, Weller C, et al. Role of chronic infection and inflammation in the gastrointestinal tract in the etiology and pathogenesis of idiopathic Parkinsonism. Part 1: eradication of Helicobacter in the cachexia of idiopathic Parkinsonism. Helicobacter Aug 2005;10(4): 267-275.

[62] Dobbs RJ, Dobbs SM, Weller C, et al. Helicobacter hypothesis for idiopathic Parkinsonism: before and beyond. Helicobacter Oct 2008;13(5): 309-322.

[63] de la Fuente-Fernandez R, Calne DB. Evidence for environmental causation of Parkinson's disease. Parkinsonism Relat Disord Mar 2002;8(4): 235-241.

[64] Bjarnason IT, Charlett A, Dobbs RJ, et al. Role of chronic infection and inflammation in the gastrointestinal tract in the etiology and pathogenesis of idiopathic Parkinsonism. Part 2: response of facets of clinical idiopathic Parkinsonism to Helicobacter pylori eradication. A randomized, double-blind,

placebo-controlled efficacy study. Helicobacter Aug 2005;10(4): 276-287.

[65] Qureshi GA, Qureshi AA, Devrajani BR, Chippa MA, and Syed SA. Is the deficiency of vitamin B12 related to oxidative stress and neurotoxicity in Parkinson's patients? CNS Neurol Disord Drug Targets Feb 2008;7(1): 20-27.

[66] Kuhn W, Roebroek R, Blom H, et al. Elevated plasma levels of homocysteine in Parkinson's disease. Eur Neurol Nov 1998;40(4): 225-227.

[67] Muller T, Werne B, Fowler B, Kuhn W. Nigral endothelial dysfunction, homocysteine, and Parkinson's disease. Lancet Jul 10 1999;354(9173): 126-127.

[68] Logroscino G, Gao X, Chen H, Wing A, and Ascherio A. Dietary iron intake and risk of Parkinson's disease. Am J Epidemiol Dec 15 2008;168(12): 1381-1388.

[69] Venderova K, Ruzicka E, Vorisek V, Visnovsky P. Survey on cannabis use in Parkinson's disease: subjective improvement of motor symptoms. Mov Disord Sep 2004;19(9): 1102-1106.

[70] Carroll CB, Bain PG, Teare L, et al. Cannabis for dyskinesia in Parkinson's disease: a randomized double-blind crossover study. Neurology Oct 12 2004;63(7): 1245-1250.

[71] Katzenschlager R, Evans A, Manson A, et al. Mucuna pruriens in Parkinson's disease: a double blind clinical and pharmacological study. J Neurol Neurosurg Psychiatry Dec 2004;75(12): 1672-1677.

[72] Manyam BV, Dhanasekaran M, Hare TA. Neuroprotective effects of the antiParkinson drug Mucuna pruriens. Phytother Res Sep 2004;18(9): 706-712.

[73] Misra L, Wagner H. Extraction of bioactive principles from Mucuna pruriens seeds. Indian J Biochem Biophys Feb 2007;44(1): 56-60.

[74] Tharakan B, Dhanasekaran M, Mize-Berge J, Manyam BV. Anti-Parkinson botanical Mucuna pruriens prevents levodopa induced plasmid and genomic DNA damage. Phytother Res Dec 2007;21(12): 1124-1126.

[75] Hellenbrand W, Boeing H, Robra BP, et al. Diet and Parkinson's disease. II: A possible role for the past intake of specific nutrients. Results from a self-administered food-frequency questionnaire in a case-control study. Neurology Sep 1996;47(3): 644-650.

[76] Fall PA, Fredrikson M, Axelson O, Granerus AK. Nutritional and occupational factors influencing the risk of Parkinson's disease: a case-control study in southeastern Sweden. Mov Disord Jan 1999;14(1): 28-37.

[77] Bender DA, Earl CJ, Lees AJ. Niacin depletion in Parkinsonian patients treated with L-dopa, benserazide, and carbidopa. Clin Sci (Lond) Jan 1979;56(1): 89-93.

[78] Kandinov B, Giladi N, and Korczyn AD. Smoking and tea consumption delay onset of Parkinson's disease. Parkinsonism Relat Disord Jan 2009;15(1): 41-46.

[79] Duvoisin RC, Yahr MD, Cote LD. Pyridoxine reversal of L-dopa effects in Parkinsonism. Trans Am Neurol Assoc 1969;94: 81-84.

[80] Evatt ML, Delong MR, Khazai N, Rosen A, Triche S, Tangpricha V. Prevalence of Vitamin D insufficiency in patients with Parkinson disease and Alzheimer disease. Arch Neurol Oct 2008;65(10): 1348-1352.

[81] Fernandes de Abreu DA, Eyles D, Feron F. Vitamin D, a neuro-immunomodulator: Implications for neurodegenerative and autoimmune diseases. Psychoneuroendocrinology Jun 20 2009.

[82] Invernizzi M, Carda S, Viscontini GS, Cisari C. Osteoporosis in Parkinson's disease. Parkinsonism Relat Disord Jun 2009;15(5): 339-346.

[83] Ono, K. and M. Yamada. Vitamin A potently destabilizes preformed alpha-synuclein fibrils in vitro: implications for Lewy body diseases. Neurobiol Dis 2007;25(2): 446-54.

[84] Lieberman A. An integrated approach to patient management in Parkinson's disease. Neurol Clin. 1992 May;10(2):553-65.

[85] Duvoisin RC, Yahr MD, Cote LD. Pyridoxine reversal of L-dopa effects in Parkinsonism. Trans Am Neurol Assoc 1969;94: 81-84.

[86] Campbell NR, Rankine D, Goodridge AE, Hasinoff BB, Kara M. Sinemet-ferrous sulphate interaction in patients with Parkinson's disease. Br J Clin Pharmacol Oct 1990;30(4): 599-605.